T0038333

अष्टाङ्ग योग

The Definitive Guide to
Therapeutic & Traditional

# YOGA

MANJU JOIS | GREG TEBB

The Acorn Press
Charlottetown
2021

I was introduced to Manju and Greg's teachings through workshops in Nova Scotia, Canada in 2011. I had studied Ashtanga for many years but the practice changed for me after studying with Manju and Greg. While I am drawn to the fast-paced vinyasas of the asana practice, I wasn't experiencing the other limbs of yoga. I still remember the weight that lifted off my shoulders when I realized that it was okay to use this practice therapeutically. I started to travel to see them whenever I could. Then the Covid-19 pandemic allowed for me to dig deeper into my practice with Greg as he started to teach online. I highly recommend his classes as well as any training you can do with Manju. Their teaching is brilliant and it has changed my life. I am forever grateful to them both.

Terrilee Bulger
Publisher

Text: Manju Jois & Greg Tebb
Translatons: All translations by Greg Tebb except where stated in the text.
Manju Jois: ManjuJois.com
Greg Tebb: gregtebb.com
Interior Color Photography: Ellen Silverman Photography except insets on pages 32,39.
www.ellensilverman.com
Cover photography and interior insets on page 32 and 39: Michael Booth
Editor for the press: Jennifer Graham
Sanskṛt Editor: Erik Marrero
Art Direction: Kathi Rota
Yogāsana Cikitsā Bhāga: Edited by Pauline Yoo in 2010 edition.

ACORNPRESS
PO Box 22024
Charlottetown, PE C1A9J2

Printed and Bound in Canada
AC0187

Library and Archives Canada Cataloguing in Publication
Title: The definitive guide to therapeutic & traditional yoga / Manju Jois, Greg Tebb.
Other titles: Definitive guide to therapeutic and traditional yoga
Names: Jois, Manju, author. | Tebb, Gregory, author.
Description: Includes index.
Identifiers: Canadiana 20210124318 | ISBN 9781773660523 (hardcover)
Subjects: LCSH: Aṣṭāṅga yoga. | LCSH: Aṣṭāṅga yoga—Therapeutic use.
Classification: LCC RA781.68 .J65 2021 | DDC 613.7/046—dc23

© 2021 by Manju Jois and Greg Tebb. All rights reserved. No part this book may be reproduced in any form or by any means, electronic or mechanical, without express permission from Manju Jois and Greg Tebb. No photographs in this book may be reproduced in any form or by any means, electronic or mechanical, without express permission from Manju Jois and Greg Tebb.

All rights reserved. No part of this book may be reproduced, stored in a retrieval system or transmitted in any form or by any means without prior permission or, in the case of photocopying, or other reprographic copying, permission from Access Copyright, 1 Yonge Street, Suite 1900, Toronto, Ontario, M5E 1E5.

Not all physical activity or exercise is suitable for everyone, and thus you should consult a physician before starting this or any exercise program. You should consult a healthcare professional if you have an injury or a medical condition. Nothing in this book should be considered medical advice or a substitute for medical consultation with a healthcare professional.

*For Nancy and Sathu*

*—MJ*

*For Kathi and Josh*

*—GT*

## Table of Contents

To write a book encompassing the teachings of the beloved "Guru", * Manju Jois, is no easy task. A guide to thousands, myself included, Manju (which means "sweet" in Sanskṛt) is a living, breathing bridge to authentic Eastern yoga traditions. I first met him nearly 25 years ago, and while I was introduced to yoga as a teenager in New Zealand and went on to study ballet, martial arts and massage therapy, it wasn't until working with Manju that things came together for me, and I truly understood the importance of a balanced yoga practice for health and harmony in body, mind and soul.

Like many, what first drew me to Manju was his flexible, creative and lighthearted approach which disguises a depth of knowledge accumulated from 65 years of practice. He was born into a yogic family in Mysore, India and combines ancient yoga techniques, traditional Vedic wisdom and even Āyurvedic cooking skills passed down from his mother. Manju's teachings are not static. Instead, he draws from a lifetime of postures, breathing, and Sanskṛt chanting to give his students the appropriate "recipe," to use his term, in order to advance the whole person. This commitment leads to a dynamic healthy body coupled with a deeply satisfying internal happiness.

This book reflects 20+ years of my study and apprenticeship with Manju and brings together the four main limbs of his teaching: yoga therapy, traditional vinyasa yoga, pranayama and chanting. It is my hope that all who pick up this book are similarly inspired by Manju's techniques and approach regardless of age or ability. As such, this book is broken into three parts.

The first section Yogāsana Cikitsā Bhāga outlines a number of postures, chosen by Manju, from the three traditional sequences (primary, intermediate and advanced). It shows how to apply adjustments and highlights potential medical and meditative benefits of each. In addition, it goes over the use of props to de-pressure joints in order to give access to difficult muscle ranges.

*Manju refers to himself as a guide.

In the second section readers will find the first two postural sequences of Ashtanga Yoga: Yoga Cikitsā, (primary series), and Nadī Śodhana (intermediate series), including their Sanskṛt counting method and instructions on the correct use of Sūrya Namaskāra (Sun Salutation) and its application for moving in and out of postures. This builds tremendous heat and sweat, which dramatically increases circulation and detoxifies, stabilizes and realigns the body for health, mental clarity and vibrancy.

The final section of the book delves into Prāṇāyāma (breathing exercises) and Sanskṛt chanting, both Vedic and Classical. These techniques have a calming, energizing and empowering effect on the body and mind, redirecting and redistributing energy from asana practice.

Scattered throughout the book are ancient Haṭha Yoga teachings in Sanskṛt, which provide more technical and therapeutic guidelines for postures and breathing techniques. Additional advanced postures are included to enhance strength, flexibility and provide a bridge into the advanced series, which should be learnt under the guidance of a competent teacher.

You will also notice that the models photographed in each chapter are in their 40s through 60s. They are all students with families, careers and households to juggle. What connects them is a dedication to bettering the mind, body and spirit by finding balance through yoga, which is the goal of this book.

As the sage Swātmarāma said, "Yuvā vṛddho'tivṛddho vā vyādhito durbalo'pi vā." Yoga is for the young, the old, the very old, the sick and the weak.

In other words, yoga is for everyone.

Greg Tebb
2021

# ....स्थूल सूक्षम कारनात् शरीरत् त्रताली लीन नीकलि न पुल दृष्ट पतले शवै भवो भगवान्

...Sthūla sūkṣma kāranāt śarīrat tritālī līna nīkali na pula dṛṣṭa patale śavai bhavo bhagavān

This yogic spiritual practice "...is for the sake of the body, the heavy and the overly slim, for understanding the gross and the subtle body, for sake of (merging) the three worlds into the Bud. It is not for the sake of being in the world, with the seen and the dead. It is to clean up all the problems so one is fit to be in the state of Bhagavan (God)." Traditional Vedic Chant

Translation: Manju Jois and Greg Tebb

ॐ वन्दे गुरूणां चरणारविन्दे संदर्शितस्वात्मसुखावबोधे ।
निःश्रेयसे जाङ्गलिकायामाने संसारहालाहलमोहशान्त्यै ॥

आबाहु पुरुषाकारं शङ्खचक्रासिधारिणम् ।
सहस्रशीरसं श्वेतं प्रणमामि पतञ्जलिम् ॥ ॐ ॥

Om vande gurūṇām caraṇāravinde sandarśita svātmasukhāvabodhe |
niḥśreyase jāṅgalikāyāmāne samsāra hālāhala mohaśāntyai ||

Ābāhu puruṣākāram śaṅkhacakrāsi dhāriṇam |
sahasra śīrasam śvetam praṇamāmi patañjalim || Om ||

Opening Prayer

I worship at the feet of the gurus, who show us the good knowledge, who are the jungle physicians, and who enlighten us to the poison of Samsāra, conditioned existence.

I bow down to Patañjali, who is in the shape of a man up to his shoulders, holding a conch, a discus of light, a sword and with a thousand white heads.

"You don't always have to teach in order of the series. Teach what is right for the person at the time."

Manju Jois

"The touch of the hand, the hand's massage."

Great teachers can "see" into their students. Manju's hands are like a surgeon's, finding difficult areas in his students and delicately fine-tuning them year after year.

The postures awaken the internal focus. Through this clarity comes an ability to notice those same struggles in others.

Manju also guides his students and teachers to develop their own mind's eye through the touch the hand. By placing our hands on another's body we can get a real sense of that person's "struggle." With a lot of practice the hands become very sensitive, and we start to feel where the person needs work. The most transformative tool is to awaken our sensitivity to what's impeding the body, not just the struggle itself. Then we can apply the hasta-sparśa and hasta-mardana to heal those in need.

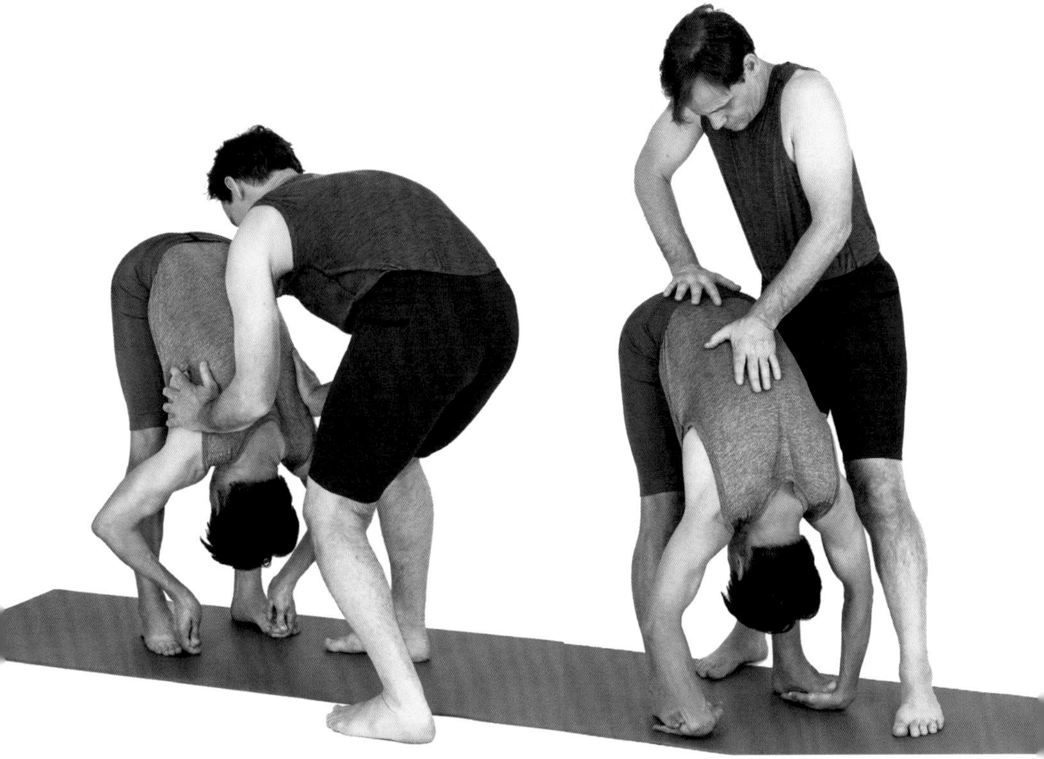

**KEY POINTS:**
The student's hips and shoulders should line up evenly, both side to side and front to back, except in the case of a leg length discrepancy (i.e., one leg is longer than another).

**ADJUSTMENT TECHNIQUES:**

1. Clasp the student's shoulder blades and draw the torso forward and down. If necessary, apply more pressure on one side to stretch the hips and buttock muscles evenly.
2. Place one hand on the sacrum area (back of the pelvis) and use the other hand to massage down the back.

**BENEFITS**:

**Muscles, Joints & Nerves:**
From these postures one receives a full stretch in the back of the body from the toes to the head. All the muscles of the back, pelvis, and legs are loosened and toned. These two postures help to rebalance the hips and pelvis. They also relieve upper body and neck tension and are helpful in curing and stabilizing issues related to the sciatic nerve, the lumbar spine, the sacrum, and problems around coccyx.

**Organs & Viscera:**
Once the student's muscular development allows access to the posture, the pelvic organs, including the bladder, prostate, reproductive system, colon, small intestine and kidneys, are invigorated.

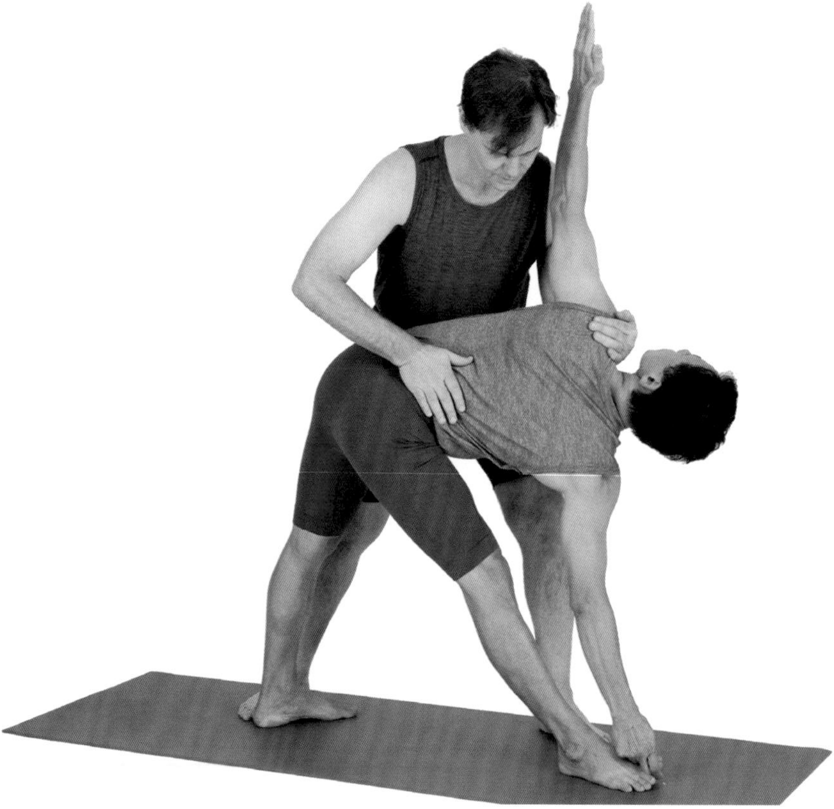

**KEY POINTS:**
The student should be balanced on both feet. In Utthita Trikoṇāsana, the torso should lined up over the front leg. In Parivṛtta Trikoṇāsana, there should be an even twist through the spine. In both postures, the upper arm should be straight up from the shoulder.

**ADJUSTMENT TECHNIQUES:**

1. Utthita Trikoṇāsana: Secure the student with your hip and place one hand on the shoulder from open/front side of the student. Massage from the base of the lower spine to the neck area.
2. Parivṛtta Trikoṇāsana: Stabilize the student with your hip and place one hand on the shoulder. Then place the other palm on on the lower spine. Massage from the base of the lower spine to the neck area.

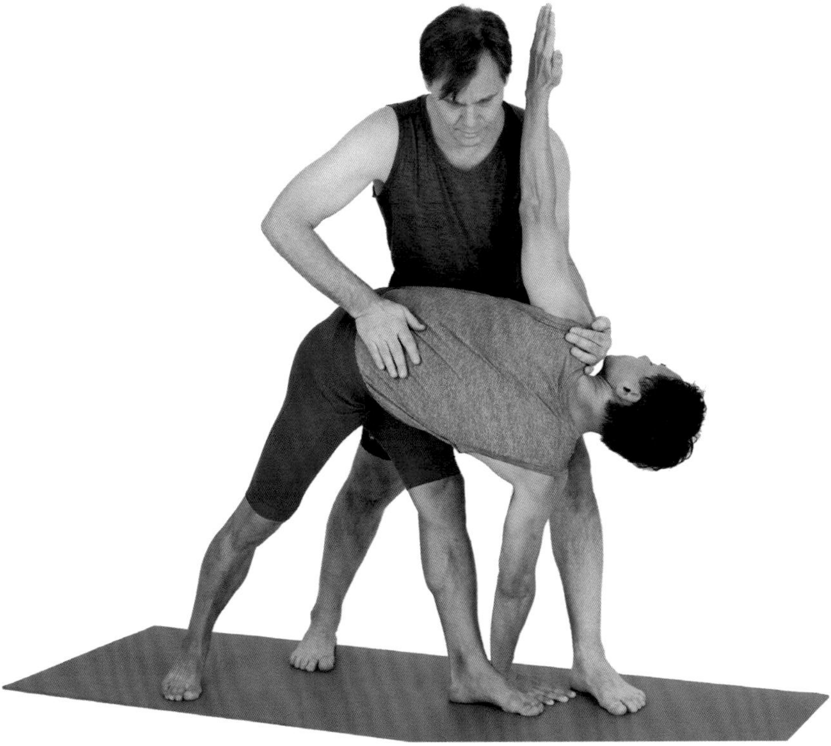

**BENEFITS:**

**Muscles, Joints & Nerves:**

Utthita Trikoṇāsana gives a full stretch to the side of body, the hips, the waist and back of ribs. It also stretches the shoulder, shoulder blade area and upper back.

Parivṛtta Trikoṇāsana additionally tones and strengthens the abdominal and spinal musculature.

**Organs & Viscera:**

Both posture variations tone and realign the lumbar spine and ribs. The areas around the lumbar nerve plexus, the femoral and sciatic nerve pathways are respaced and aligned. This helps to alleviate sciatic nerve pain in the back of the legs and gives better functionality to the all the leg muscles.

With the compression created in the Parivṛtta variation, the digestive system is rejuvenated and made stronger. Through the resetting and toning of the diaphragm and intercostal muscles, the lungs are made to function better. The hip socket area (Nitamba Marma) is clarified giving access to the base of spine (Gudam Marma) which energizes those two areas as well as the spine.

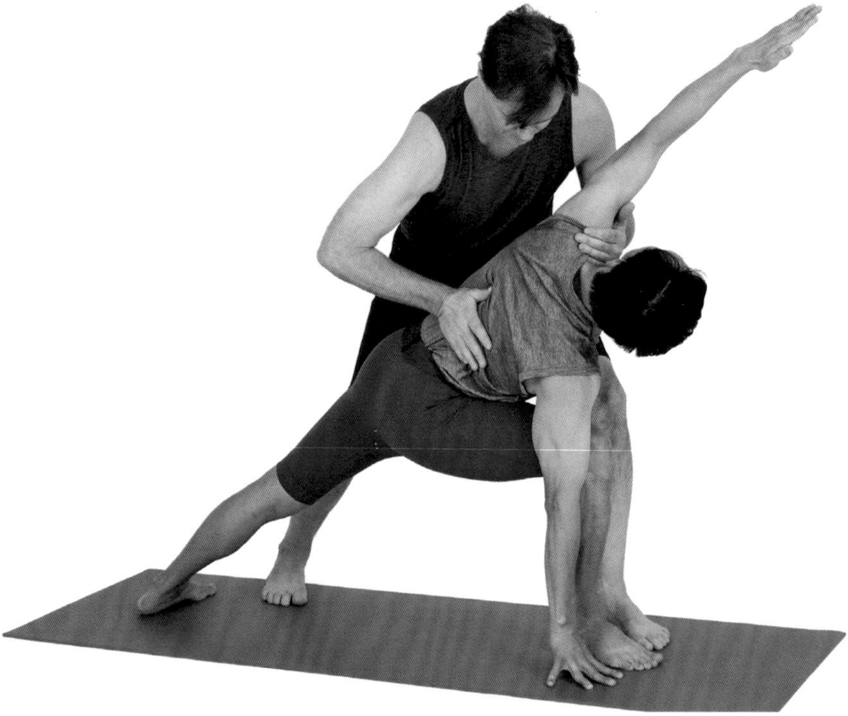

**KEY POINTS:**

The student should have a complete stretch of the side of body. There should be a full stretch in the top arm through the shoulder blade, wrist, and fingers, and the arm should be placed close to the side of the head. The arm close to the knee and foot should have a relaxed placement.

**ADJUSTMENT TECHNIQUES:**

Utthita Pārśva Koṇāsanam: Stand on the open/front side and secure the student with your hip and your hand (on the student's shoulder). Massage from the base of lower spine to the shoulder area.

Parivṛtta Pārśva Koṇāsanam: Secure the student with your hip and place your palm on the student's lower rib area. Massage from the base of lower spine to the shoulder area.

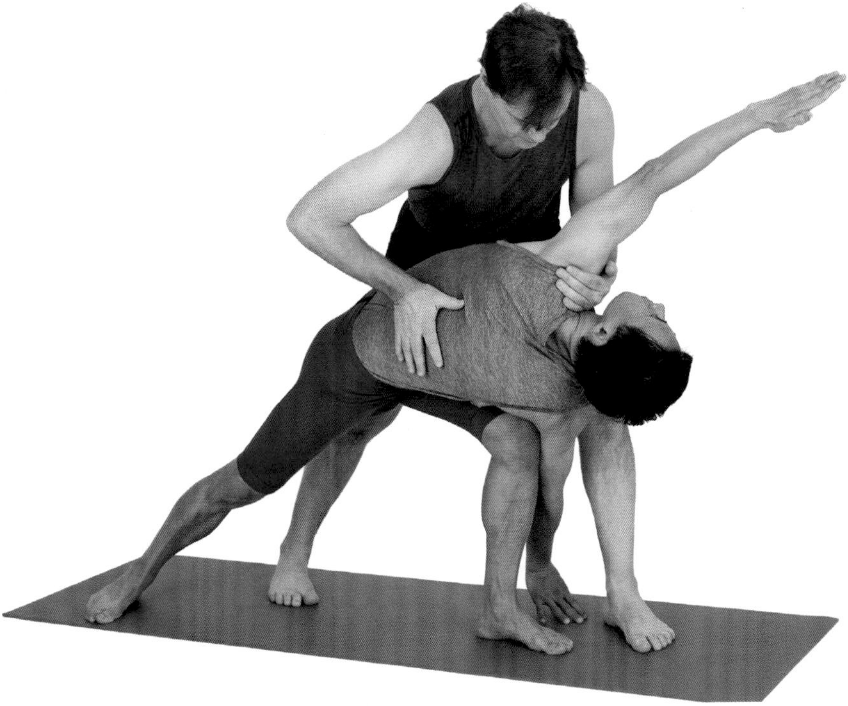

**BENEFITS:**

**Muscles, Joints & Nerves:**

These variations fully stretch and tone the side areas and muscles of the body and strengthen the legs. In particular, the tensor fascia latae (also known as the IT band) is lengthened to relieve pain in the area (side of thigh). The muscles of the back surrounding the spine are allowed greater freedom of movement. Tension is relieved in and around the lumbar vertebrae which helps free up compression on lumbar discs. The arm placement facilitates the loosening of the shoulder blade and side rib area. This can relieve pressure in the rotator cuff area, (the shoulder and shoulder-blade muscular attachments) and help achieve optimal shoulder and arm functionality.

**Organs & Viscera:**

By these two postures, the colon area (in particular, the ascending and descending colon) is alternately compressed and lengthened and stimulated, which helps correct the natural functioning of the bowel. Diet is also a key ingredient to proper bowel function. Rib muscle tension is reduced leading to the greater expansion of chest, lungs and movement of the diaphragm.

Parivṛtta Pārśva Koṇāsanam tones and invigorates all the abdominal organs. The side fascial connection from the ankle to the neck, which corresponds to the gallbladder and kidneys meridian line from Chinese medicine, is fully stretched. Also, this posture combined with Urdhva and Adho Mukha Śvānāsana stretches and prepares the ankle and energizes the Gulpa (ankle) Marma, which helps energize the feet and ankles.

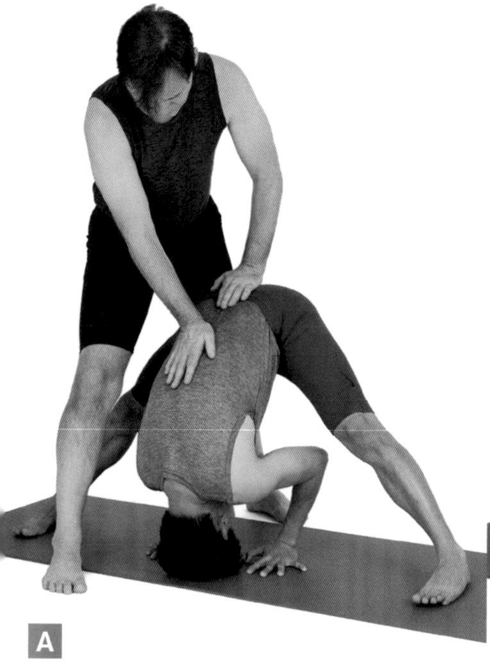


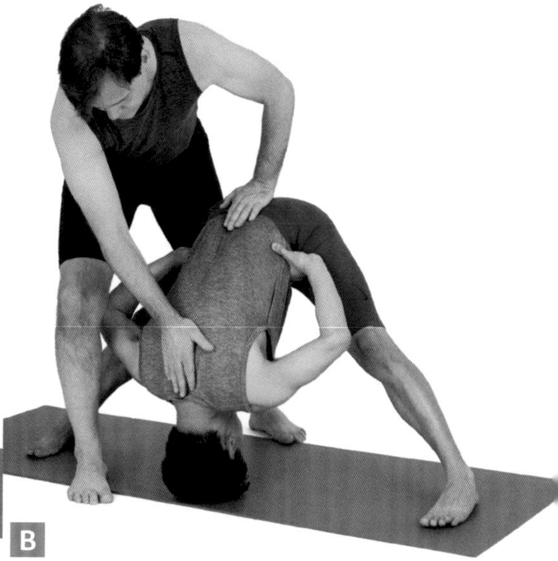


**KEY POINTS:**
Equal stretch on both hips and equal weight on both feet. The head should rest on the floor (not pressed down, but as if a piece of paper could slide under with the crown of the head and floor).

**ADJUSTMENT TECHNIQUES:**
Variations A, B, and D (Prathama, Dwitīya, and Caturtha): Straddle one leg of the student. Then place one palm on the sacrum area and one hand at the base of the spine. Massage the spine toward the head.

**Variation C (Tṛtīya):**
Stand with both legs in the front of the student's body. Then with one hand hold the student's hands and with the other hold the neck and upper back area. Massage the neck/upper back area to facilitate release in the shoulders, neck, upper back and chest muscles.

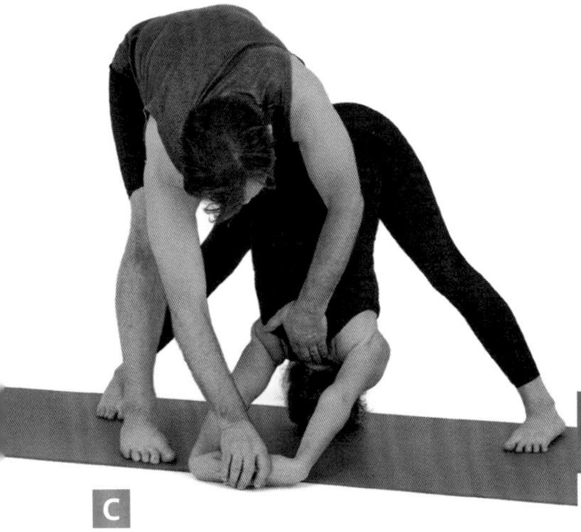

C

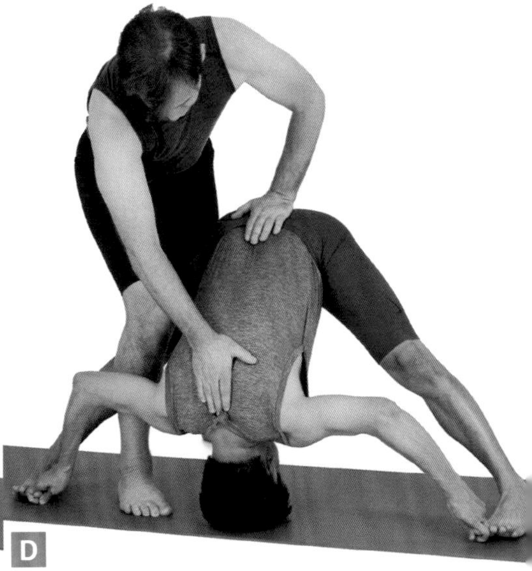

D

**BENEFITS:**

**Muscles, Joints & Nerves:**

These variations balance and stretch all the leg muscles, and in particular, the adductor and abductor muscles. The variations of this posture also can relieve sciatica nerve pain into the legs. Further, they help prepare students for inverted postures. Once the student's head can rest on the floor, facial and neck tension can be felt and relaxed. The posture also relieves muscle tension, which can inhibit the circulation to the nerves in the head and face (cervical and cranial nerves).

**Variation C (Tṛtīya):** clears tension from the upper back, neck and throat (Viśuddhi Cakra). It relieves the body of tension felt from the shoulders through the occipital area (back of the head). It helps restore the natural movement in the arms, shoulders, chest, upper back and neck muscles (in particular the Deltoid, Trapezius, Rhomboids, Pectoralis muscles, Splenius Cervicis, and Capitis).

**Organs & Viscera:**

These postures tone and rebalance all the organs of pelvis. The detensioning of the ribs and back muscles leads to better breathing and lung expansion. The inverted aspect of the poses can relieve head, facial and chest tension, which is helpful in alleviating tension headaches and eye strain.

**Variation C (Tṛtīya):** energizes the Nikanta Marma in the throat pit (supra sternal notch, important for breathing excersises).

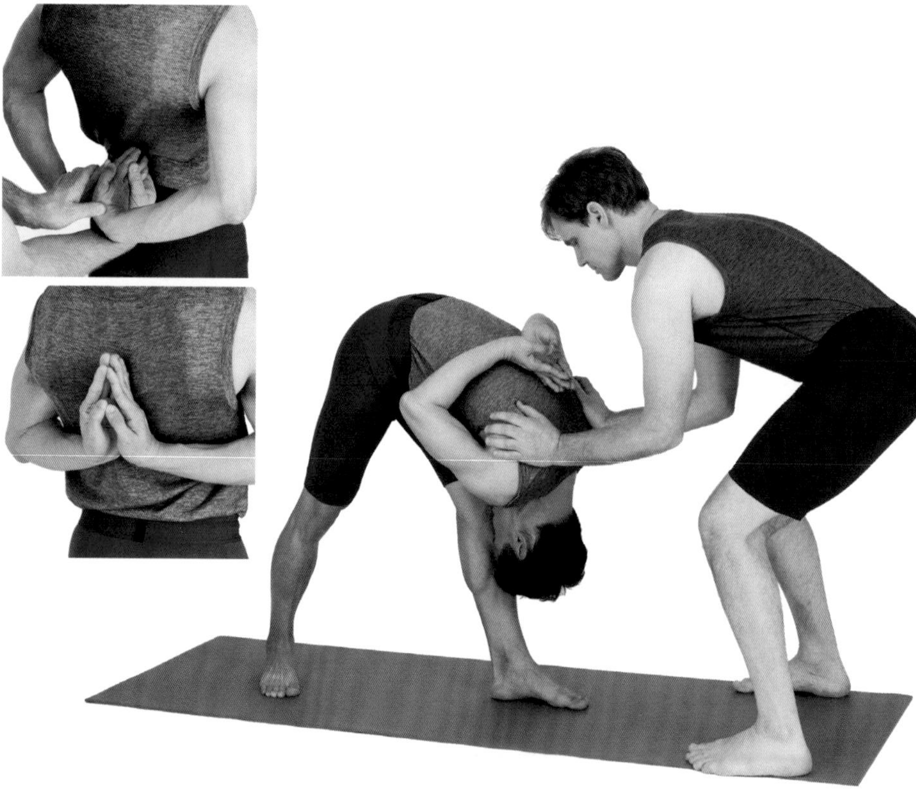

**KEY POINTS:**
The heels should line up, the legs should be straight, and the head should rest in a relaxed position on the leg. The palms of the hands should be between the shoulder blades.

**ADJUSTMENT TECHNIQUES:**
Place both hands on the student's shoulder blades by gripping the side of the shoulder blade area. Then press the student's chest toward the leg.

**BENEFITS:**

**Muscles, Joints & Nerves:**
This posture gives a full stretch to the open side of the body. It rebalances pelvic and hip muscles and ensures functional movement in the sacroiliac (back of pelvis) joint. It tones the legs, abdominal and back muscles. The shoulders, neck, chest, and upper back areas are nicely stretched. This posture can be very helpful for lower back nerve and disc issues.

**Organs & Viscera:**
Once the posture is mastered, it tones the breathing musculature and thereby benefits the lungs. The kidneys and bladder are invigorated through compression and deep stretching. The variation clarifies the specific lines of stretch relating to the heart, lung, intestines, kidneys and bladder. The stretch of the connections from the hips to ribs stimulates and supports praṇic energy in the chest and apāna energy in the anus. This in turn stimulates the Jaṭhara Agni (digestive fire).

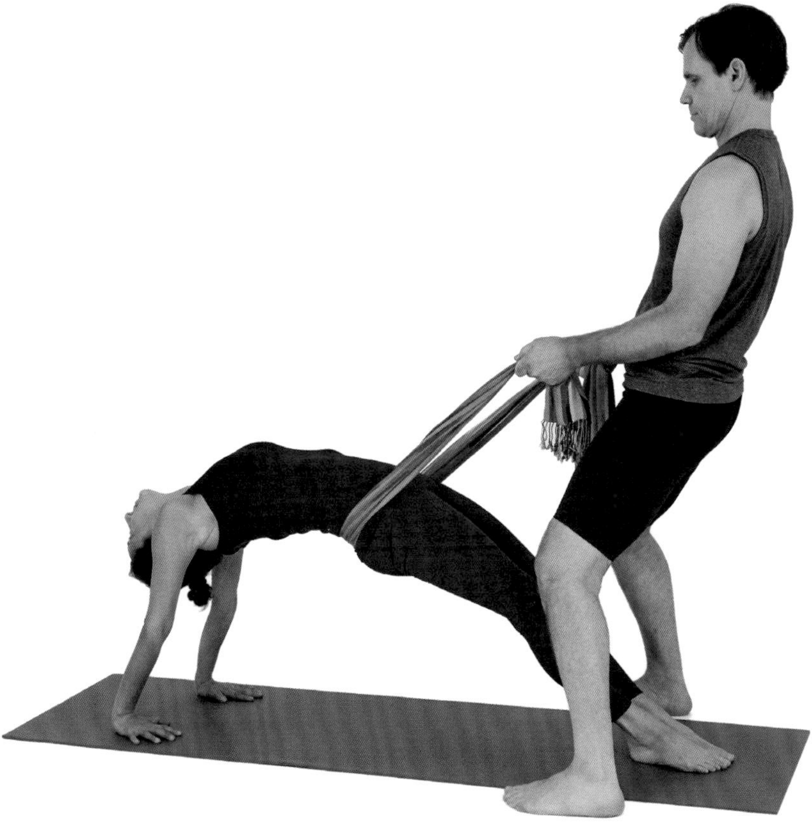

**KEY POINTS:**
This posture is a long stretch through the front body from the toes to the chin. Ideally, it is performed with no bend in the knees. The arms should be placed shoulder width.

**ADJUSTMENT TECHNIQUES:**
Place a strap around the back of the student's hips and pull the strap diagonally "through" the pelvis to create the lift required to complete the curve through the front of body.

**BENEFITS:**

**Muscles, Joints & Nerves:**
One receives a full stretch from toes to chin and a corresponding strengthening of all the back of the body. Once the flexibility of the posture is gained, the upper back and shoulders receive a tremendous workout.

**Organs & Viscera:**
The pelvic floor is strengthened and is a boon for strengthening the perineal and anal area, and for toning and invigorating the whole genital and pelvic area. The tissue surrounding the female reproductive system is stretched and strengthened. The bladder is reenergized and the viscera surrounding the bladder meridian is clarified through the stretch. The digestive system is stretched; one often hears the movement of fluid in the colon when the full stretch is applied from the pelvis through the ribs. The posture stimulates the Vipata Marma, energizing the whole pelvic area.

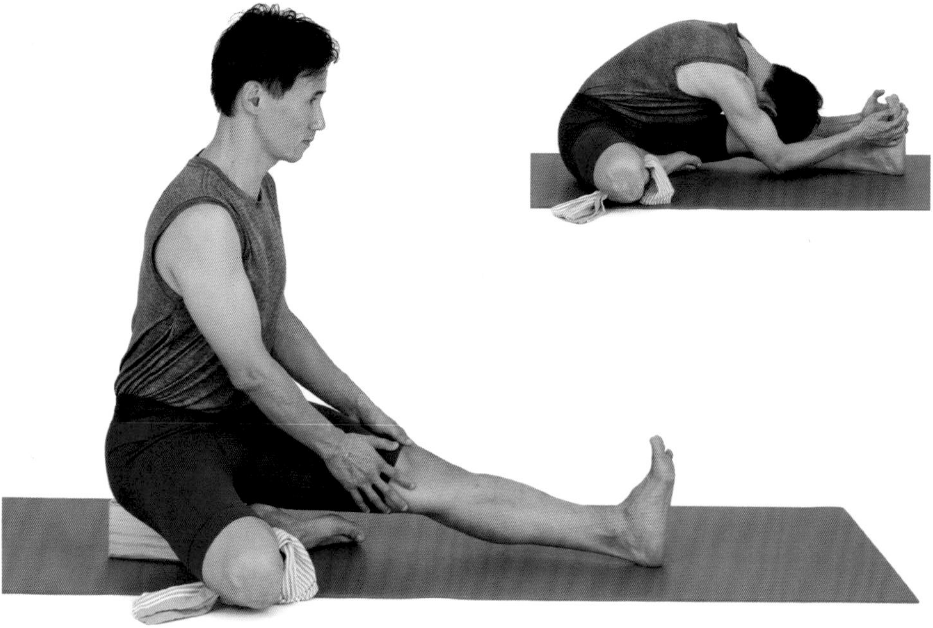

**KEY POINTS:**
The front leg is stretched, and the other leg is bent with the heel pressed close into the groin. After a forward bend the head should rest on the knee or shin of the outstretched leg.

**MODIFICATION:**
If the student has knee problems, they can place a towel in the back of the bent knee, or sit on a block to create space for the joint.

**BENEFITS:**
**Muscles, Joints & Nerves:**
The open side of the body receives a deep stretch into the hip and buttock area. The lower spine and side ribs are fully opened and stretched. This posture is usually a therapeutic variation for those with lower back problems and sciatic nerve issues.

**Organs & Viscera:**
According to Swātmārāma, this posture has tremendous benefits and cures many diseases in the abdominal and upper spinal area, including lung problems. This variation and Jānu Śīrṣāsanam B (dwitīya) can help those suffering from problems around the anal area.

क्षयकुष्ठगुदावर्त्तगुल्माजीर्णपुरोगमाः।
तस्य दोषाः क्षयं यान्ति महामुद्रां तु योऽभ्यसेत् ॥ ३:१७ ॥

Kṣayakuṣṭhagudādarttagulmājīrṇapurogamāḥ |
tasya doṣāḥ kṣayam yāntimahāmudrām tu yo'bhyaset || 3:17 ||

"From the practice of Mahāmudra (janū-śirṣāsana) there is relief from spleen or abdominal enlargement, digestive problems and diseases like Tuberculosis, Leprosy, & Piles."
HAṬHA YOGA PRAḌĪPIKĀ 3:17

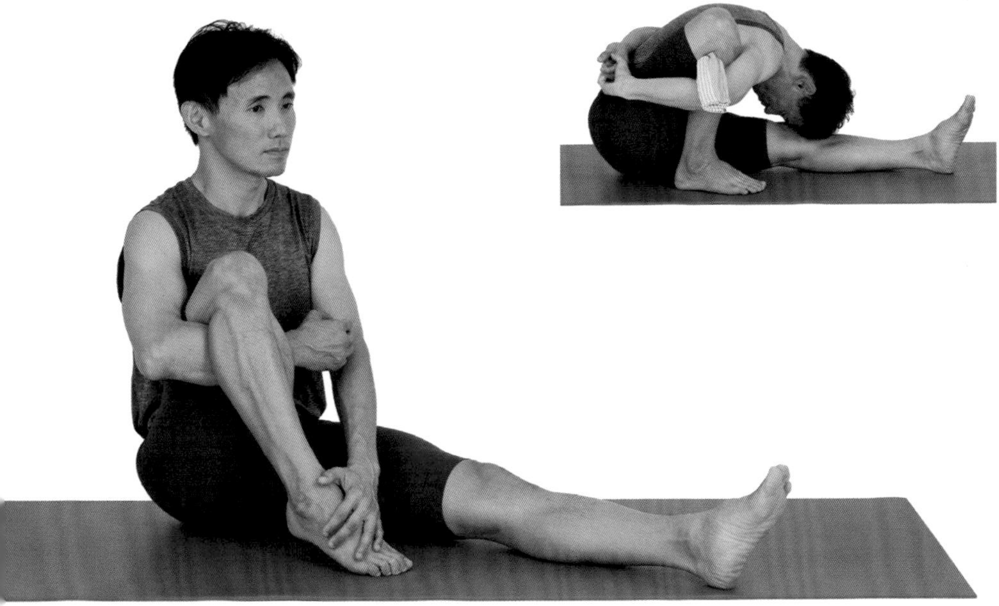

**KEY POINTS:**
The front leg is outstretched. The heel of the bent knee is close to the hip and the arm is bound around the shin of the bent knee. The spine should be relaxed so the head rests on the outstretched leg or upper shin.

**MODIFICATION:**
A cloth or towel can be placed at the back of the bent knee if there are any knee problems.

**BENEFITS:**

**Muscles, Joints & Nerves:**
These Marīcyāsana variations (A,B,C,and D--only A is photographed) have many of the same benefits of the previous forward bends. The combination of Jānu Śīrṣāsana and Marīcyāsana creates a complete stretch of the back, hips and back pelvic muscles. The many angles for stretching the shoulders and upper back alleviate rotator cuff issues (shoulder and shoulder blade trauma) and can cure subluxations (displaced vertebrae) in the cervical spine. Lower (lumbar) spinal issues are helped. The rib attachments into the thoracic spine are articulated thereby helping to restore natural movement into the back muscles and central nervous system. This posture has a regenerative effect over the whole spine.

**Organs & Viscera:**
The Marīcyāsana variations help lung function and breathing problems caused by stiffness in the diaphragm and ribcage. The posture clarifies the fascial (connective tissue) containing the heart, lung, large and small intestine meridians. The digestive system is squeezed and pressured from the forward bend, the different foot placements in Marīchyasana B, C, and D, and twisting movements, benefiting all the abdominal organs.

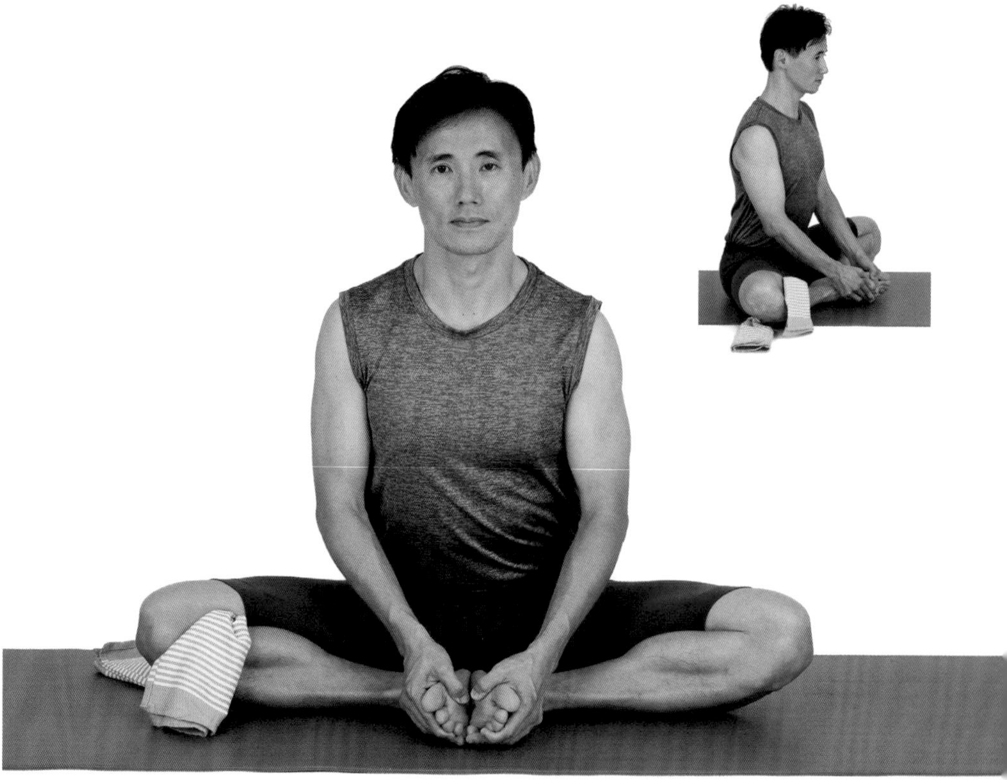

**KEY POINTS:**
The back should be straight and head held erect. The heels need to be drawn as close as possible to the groin.

**BENEFITS:**
**Muscles, Joints & Nerves:**
From the three variations (upright, forward bend, head to feet), one receives a deep stretch from the coccyx to the forehead. The hips are fully articulated and the spinal and abdominal muscles are strengthened and stretched.

**Organs & Viscera:**
As Vāmana Ṛṣi states in the commentary below, the posture plays a pivotal role for the health of the base of the spine. The muscles, nervous system and organs close to anal area are clarified, strengthened and invigorated.

बद्धकोनासने तिष्टं गुदमकुञ्चयेत् बुद्ध ।
गुदरोग्निवृत्तिः स्यात् सत्यं सत्यं ब्रविम्यहं ॥ वामन ऋषि ॥

Baddhakonāsane tiṣṭan gudamakuñcayet buddha |
gudarognivṛttiḥ syāt satyam satyam bravimyaham ||

"The wise one should retract the anus while in Baddha Koṇāsana as it wards off anal disease, this I declare is true." VĀMANA ṚṢI

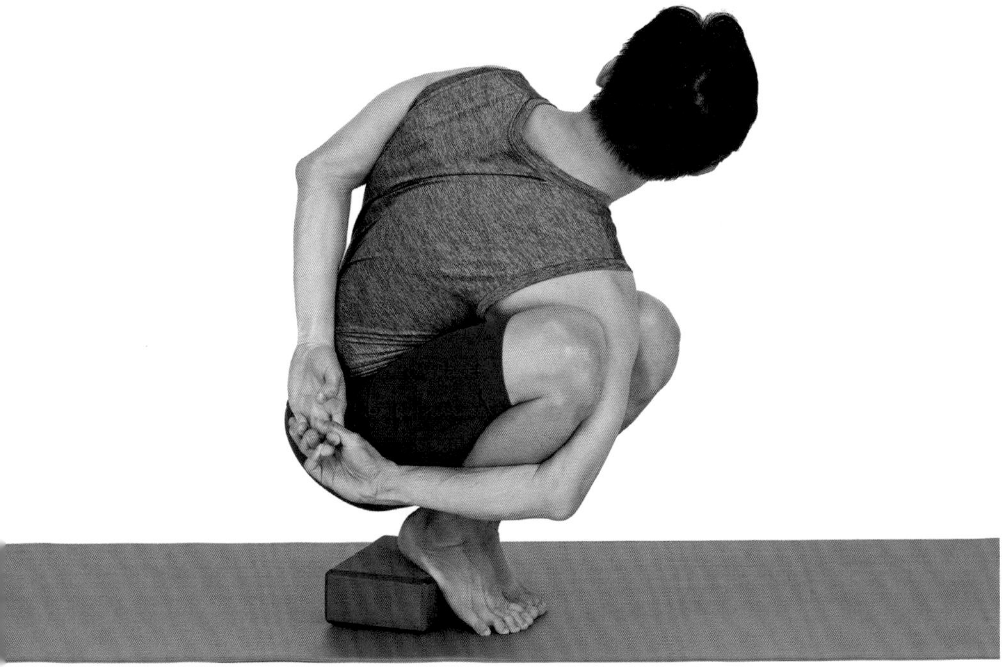

**KEY POINTS:**
The feet are fully grounded with the hands bound.

**MODIFICATIONS:**
Pāśāsana can be difficult on the knees. Swelling, arthritis, and/or knee replacements can place limitations on full flexion (folding) of the knees. A stool, low chair or block under the heels can be used to aid balance. This also allows better access to the spinal twist by relieving direct pressure on the knees. A strap can also be used for the bind if the hands do not touch.

**BENEFITS:**

**Muscles, Joints & Nerves:**
The posture strengthens the front of the legs (shins and thighs) and fully stretches the ankles and plantar muscles of the feet. The spinal muscles receive a deep stretch and all the abdominal and spinal muscles are toned. Pāśāsana can be helpful for lower back problems such as sciatica and compression in the lumbar spine. It is also beneficial for athletes and runners suffering from ankle stiffness, shin splints, plantar fascia problems, and lower-leg cramps.

**Organs & Viscera:**
Pāśāsana tones the digestive system and invigorates all the organs of the pelvis. The musculature for breathing (intercostal muscles, inferior and superior posterior serratus and the diaphragm) is toned leading to deeper breathing and stimulating better lung function.

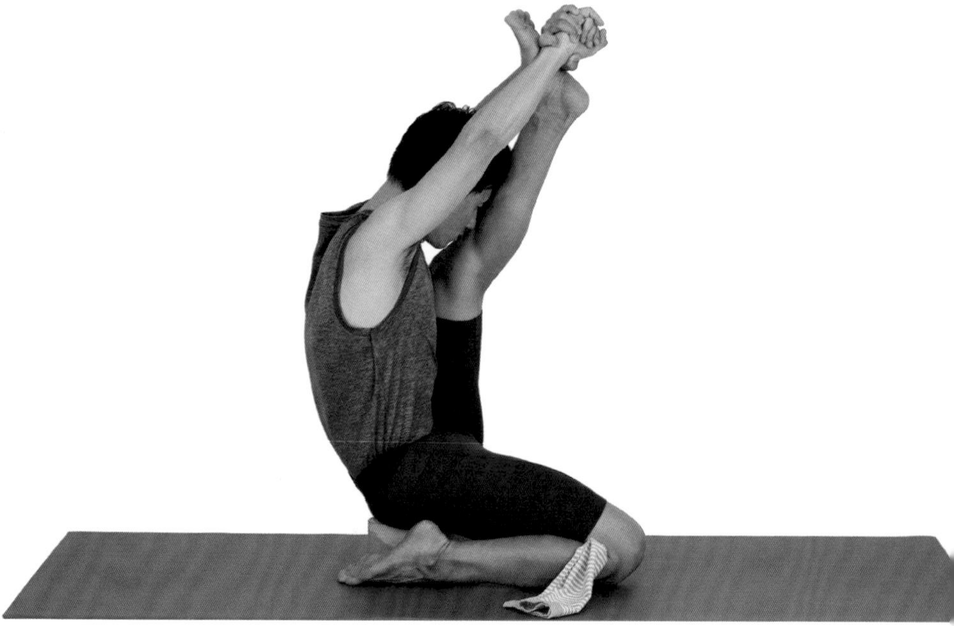

**KEY POINTS:**
Both hips should be on the floor. One leg is extended straight and raised in front of the torso. The other leg is tucked beside the hip with the knee bent. The head should rest on the raised extended leg with the arms binding the foot of the extended leg.

**MODIFICATION:**
The heel of the extended leg can be placed on the floor close to the sit bone (ischial tuberosity) instead of being stretched upward. This posture is an advanced version of Tiryañc Mukhaikapāda Paścimatānāsana in Primary Series. If the student has any difficulty with that posture, then modifications with a block under the hip and/or cloth behind the knee can be helpful.

**BENEFITS:**
**Muscles, Joints & Nerves:**
The muscles on the back of the extended leg receive a full stretch. When the knee is placed correctly on the floor, the front (quadriceps) of the bent leg and shin muscles (tibialis anterior and toe extensors) receive a full stretch. The posture relieves tension in the pathway of the femoral and sciatic nerves and thereby helps to improve the health and optimal functioning of all the leg muscles. The nervous system around the sacrum and coccyx is stretched and rebalanced.

**Organs & Viscera:**
This posture invigorates both the male and female reproductive systems. The ascending, descending and sigmoid areas of the colon receive a massage and thus helps with elimination. Diet also plays a crucial role in colon health. The bladder and prostate areas are toned and energized.

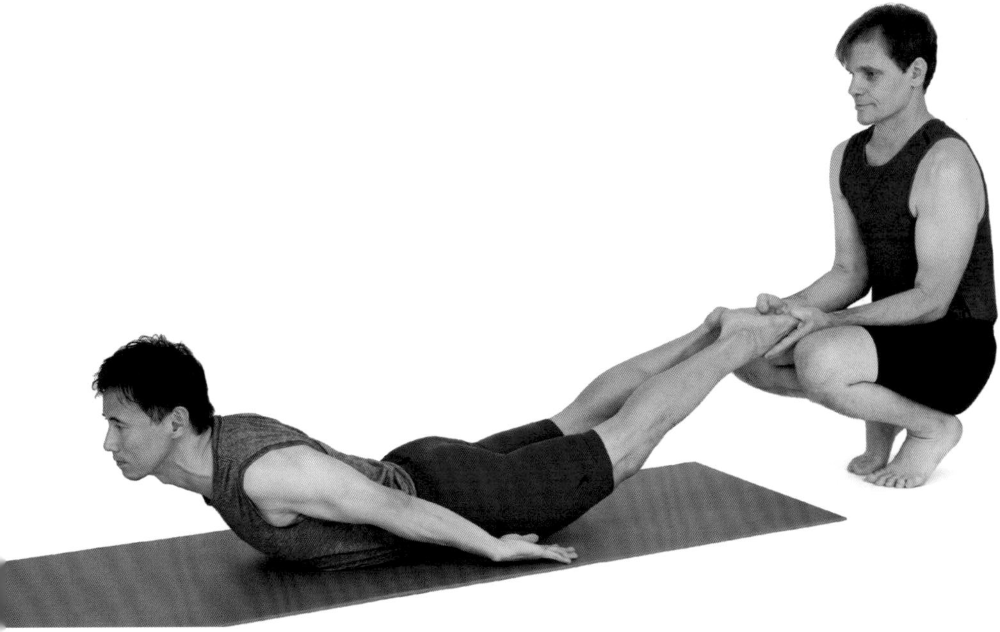

**KEY POINTS:**
Students should perform this posture with straight legs and feet close together.

**MODIFICATION:**
To the untrained body, this posture can be difficult and sometimes painful. If the lower back muscles are untrained or stiff, then one leg at a time can be lifted as a variation.

**ADJUSTMENT TECHNIQUES:**
Lengthen the student's legs to help provide the lift and knee stretch.

**BENEFITS:**

**Muscles, Joints & Nerves:**
This posture makes all the back muscles engage simultaneously. In most cases, it is beneficial for back pain, especially in the lower spine, and for sciatic nerve issues. It is particularly helpful for runners, as it stretches the psoas/hip flexor muscles.

**Organs & Viscera:**
The posture tones the digestive system and stretches the diaphragm and rib muscles to allow for deeper breathing and lung expansion. A correct stretch in Śalabhāsana invigorates the bladder through pelvic pressure and clarifies the bladder meridian. This posture stimulates Vipata and Basti Marmas which are central to pelvic energetic health.

अध्यास शेते करयुग्मवक्ष आलम्भ्य भूमि करयोस्तलाभ्याम् ।
पादौ च शुन्ये च वितस्ति चोर्ध्वम् वदन्ति पीठं शलभं मुनीन्द्राः॥ २:३९ ॥

"Lay down in a sleeping position (on stomach) hands by the chest with both palms resting on the floor. The legs are extended into the void (above the body) lifted the height of Vitasti (the extended length between tip of thumb and little finger).This is called by the sages Śalabha the locust."

GHERAṆḌA SAMHITA 2:39

TRANSLITERATION ON PAGE 91

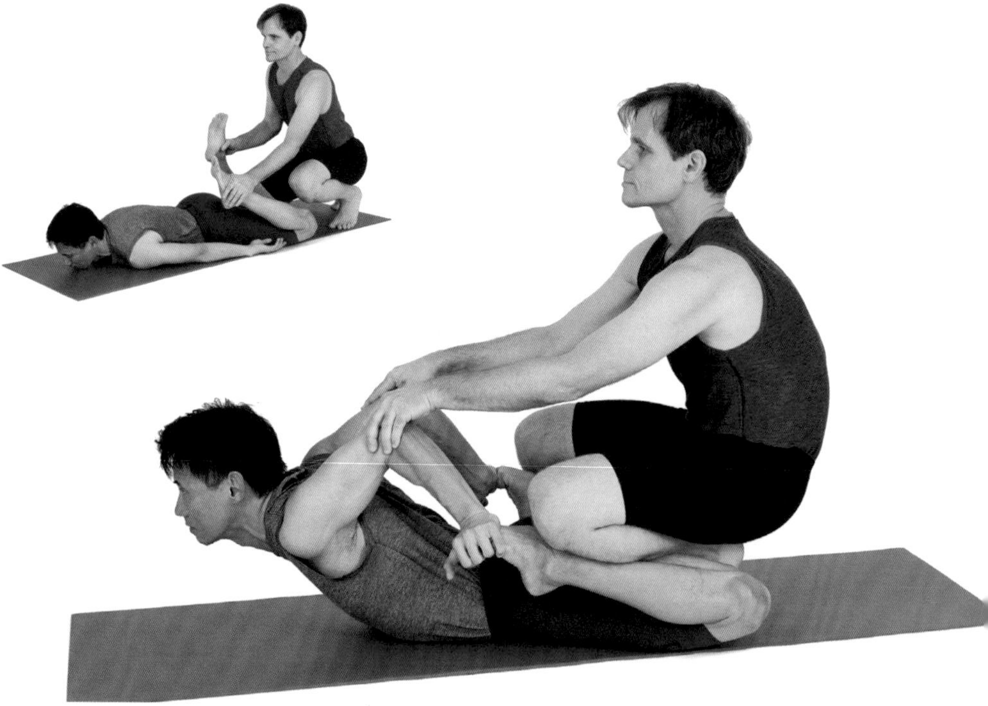

**KEY POINTS:**

The feet should be close to the hips and the heels pressed to or towards the floor. Elbows should be drawn back and the chest lifted. The heels need to be close to the hips to avoid excess strain on the knee.

**ADJUSTMENT TECHNIQUES:**

The adjuster can alternately stretch each leg by pressing the student's feet down one at a time close to the hip and towards the floor.

**BENEFITS:**

**Muscles, Joints & Nerves:**

The knee joint becomes fully flexible (in flexion). The posture encourages excess fluid around the knee to drain from the area. Also, the back muscles are strengthened and prepared for deeper bends.

This posture stretches the hips, thighs, front pelvis, and whole front torso. Additionally, the posture applies deep pressure to the pelvis, sacrum and coccyx, and thereby facilitating the natural movement and toning of these areas.

**Organs & Viscera:**

The posture opens the diaphragm to provide the abdominal cavity a deep stretch and facilitates the correct functioning of all the abdominal organs. In addition, the major breathing muscles are strengthened to give deeper access to the lungs and chest area. The posture relieves tension in both the male and female reproductive systems.

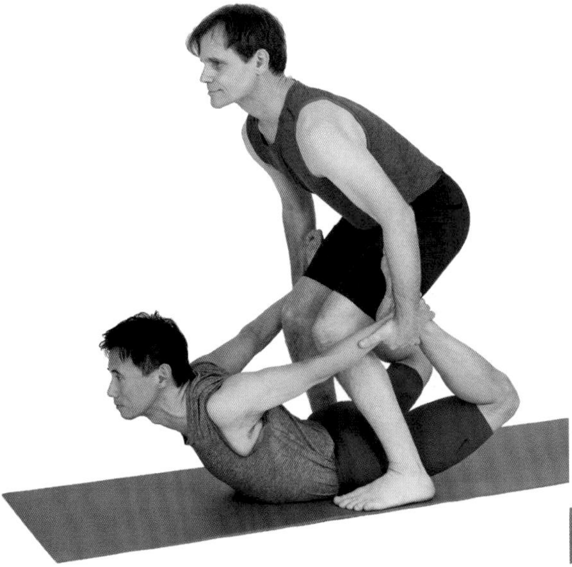

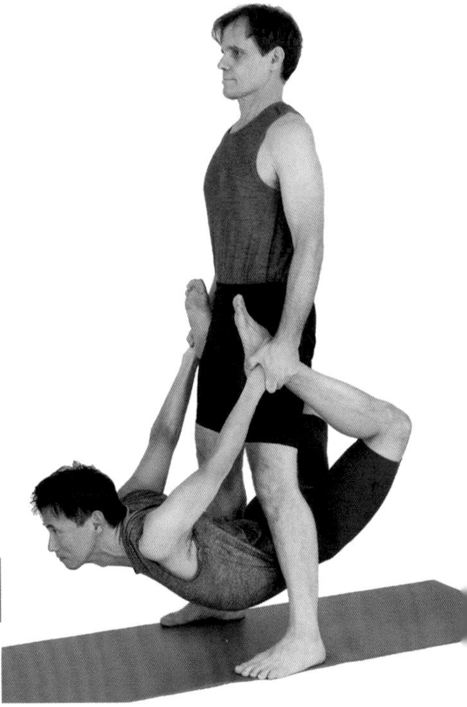

**KEY POINTS:**

The śloka on page 30 refers to the advanced version of the posture, Pādāṅguṣṭha Dhanurāsana, in which the big toes are held and brought to the ears. However, in Dhanūrasana students need only to hold the feet and stretch them to the ceiling with straight arms. The knees can be drawn together as a final variation; however, this is difficult and not always appropriate for those with lower spine issues.

**ADJUSTMENT TECHNIQUES:**

The pictured adjustment is liberating for the spine. It should not be used on those with nerve or disc problems without proper supervision and training.

Place your own feet close to the student's hips, and while bending your knees, clasp the student's ankles and wrists. Then straighten your knees while firmly holding the student's ankles and wrists. If you need more height to lift the student, you should clasp your hands together and use your forearms under the student's legs to lift.

**BENEFITS:**

**Muscles, Joints & Nerves:**

The posture provides a full stretch from the upper torso through the pelvis and into the legs. The full frontal stretch articulates the ribs and the chest muscles. By freeing the space where the ribs meet the spine both anteriorly and posteriorly, it provides a feeling of lightness, freedom and access to the diaphragm. In addition, one gets a deeper understanding of backbending and the articulation of the ribcage in relation to the spine.

**Organs & Viscera:**

The abdominal organs benefit from the deep stretch and by being pressured on the floor. This posture intensifies the work into the back muscles and goes deeper than Śalabhāsana and Bhekāsana.

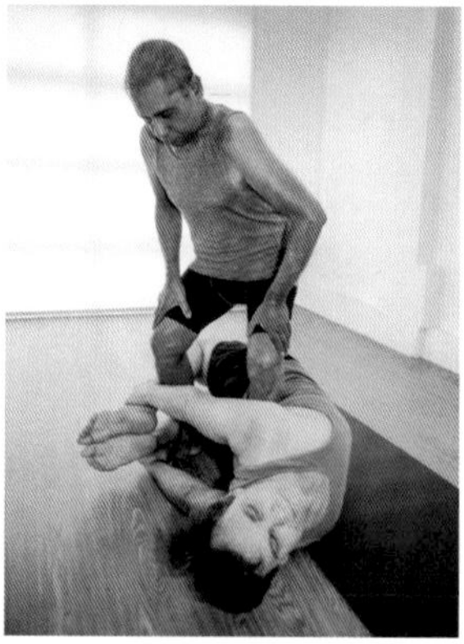

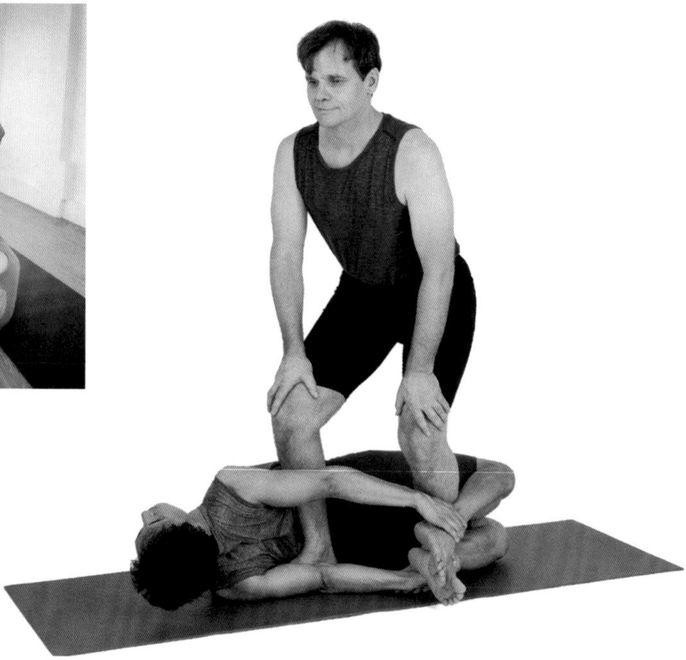

**KEY POINTS:**
The side of the body should fully touch the floor and the gaze should be up towards the ceiling. When the adjustment is applied for the bow/spinal stretch, the gaze should be neutral.

**ADJUSTMENT TECHNIQUES:**
The student should be relaxed and move with the adjustment. When the student is on his/her side, step between the student's arms and shins. Place the outside of your calf muscle against the student's back mid-ribs and calf muscles. Then stretch the student by pressing your knees apart.

**BENEFITS:**

**Muscles, Joints & Nerves:**
This posture is very similar to the Dhanurāsana except it targets the pressure of the bend more to the upper side body. The posture helps to free up the shoulders, arms, and collarbones. By resting the shape on the floor, it helps the student relax and stretch the abdominal muscles more effectively.

**Organs & Viscera:**
The adjustment applies an equal force to the ribs and lower spine and effectively articulates the thoracic spine. This frees the body to stretch the inside of the ribs and access the organs there: the lungs, heart and stomach.

पादांगुष्टौ तु पाणिभ्यां गृहीत्वा श्रवणावधि । धनुराकर्षणं कुर्याद् धनुरासनमुच्यते ॥ १:२५ ॥

Pādāṅguṣṭau tu pāṇibhyām gṛhītvā śravaṇāvadhi dhanurākarṣaṇam
kuryād dhanurāsanamucayate || 1:25 ||

"With both hands grasp the toes and bring them to the ears.
Having drawn tight the bow it is called Dhanurāsana." HAṬHA YOGA PRADĪPIKĀ 1:25

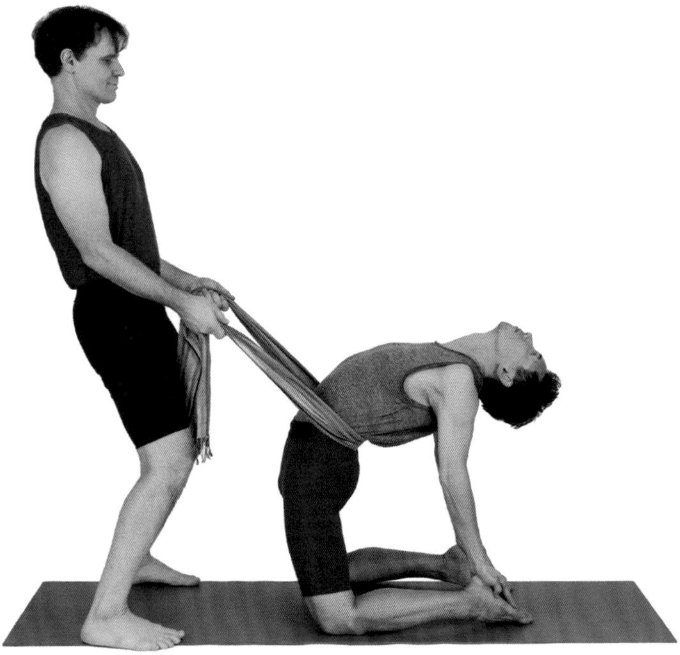

**KEY POINTS:**
Students should have the knees hip width apart and their hands reaching back and placed on the feet. They should have a relaxed and even stretch in the legs, chest, and belly.

**ADJUSTMENT TECHNIQUES:**
Stand in front of the student placing a cloth behind the student's sacrum/lower back area and lower the student into position. If the student is comfortable in the posture's full position, then a further adjustment can be given by moving the cloth up the back closer to the lower rib area.

**BENEFITS:**

**Muscles, Joints & Nerves:**
This posture stretches, lengthens, and tones the front of the legs, the stomach, and chest muscles. It also helps develop the deeper backbends. The posture clarifies the nerve pathways to the arms and legs (lumbar and brachial plexus) as well as the accompanying muscles and fascia (connective tissue) from the feet to the throat and from the palm to the chest.

**Organs & Viscera:**
Uṣṭrāsana improves the health and vitality of the digestive system. By loosening and toning the diaphragm, chest, and intercostal muscles, the posture improves lung power and breath capacity. This in turn gives space and access to the bronchial tubes. The postures applies a wonderful stretch to the pelvis, the bladder area, and genitals, and revitalizes the whole area.

अध्यास्य शेते पदयुग्मव्यस्तं पृष्ठे निधायापि धृतं कराभ्याम् ।
आकुंच्य सम्यग्ध्युदरास्यगधं उष्ट्रश्च पीठं यतयो वदन्ति॥ २:४१ ॥

"Place the feet down in the "sleeping position" (on the floor) even and separated. Bring the hands to the feet then intensely stretch of the belly. This is called Uṣtra (camel) seat by the sages."

GHERAṆḌA SAMHITA 2:41

TRANSLITERATION ON PAGE 94

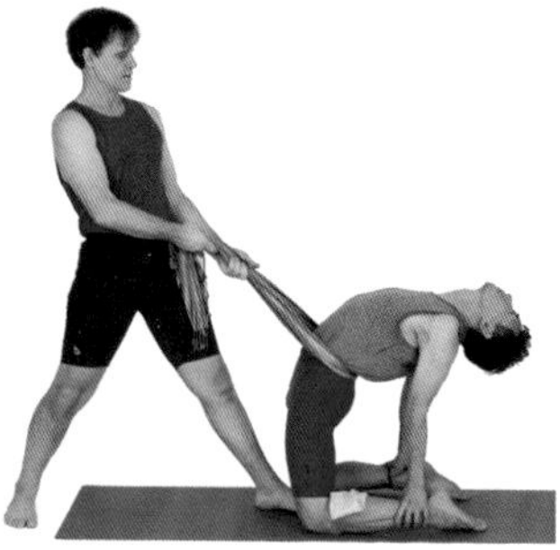

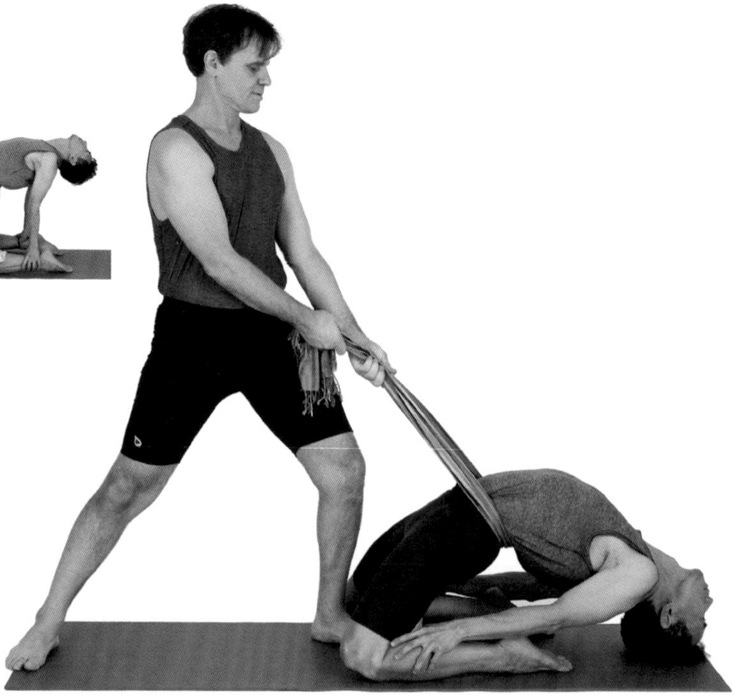

**KEY POINTS:**
The posture is a variation of Uṣṭrāsana. The hips and arms should remain fully stretched. The hands are placed on the ankles with the elbows stretched throughout the posture.

**ADJUSTMENT TECHNIQUES:**
Place the strap on top of the student's sacral area and stand firmly in front of the student with both feet secured and a straight back. As you lower the student's head to the floor, lean back and maintain good posture.

**BENEFITS:**

**Muscles, Joints & Nerves:**
In addition to the benefits of Uṣṭrāsana, this posture strengthens the torso, quadriceps, inner thighs, and pelvic muscles. This is a fundamental posture for developing the third variation of these postures, Kapotāsana.

**Organs & Viscera:**
This posture provides a boost to the musculature around the coccyx and sacrum, and stimulates the nerves of the surrounding tissues and organs.

**मेरुदण्डग्रन्थिदोर्ढ्यंसंपिपादयिषुः पुमान् ।**
**कपोतोष्ट्रासनाभ्यासं कुर्यान्मितहियाशनः ॥ योग रहस्य २:२१ ॥**

Merudaṇḍagranthidordhyamsampipādayishuḥ pumān |
kapotoṣtrāsanābhyāsam kuryānmitahiyāśanaḥ || 2.21 ||

"For the man who desires firmness or stability in the spine and grathis (yogic knots of the spine) they should practice Uṣtrāsana and Kapotāsana (3rd deeper variation). One should also eat a moderate and suitable diet." YOGA RAHASYA 2:21

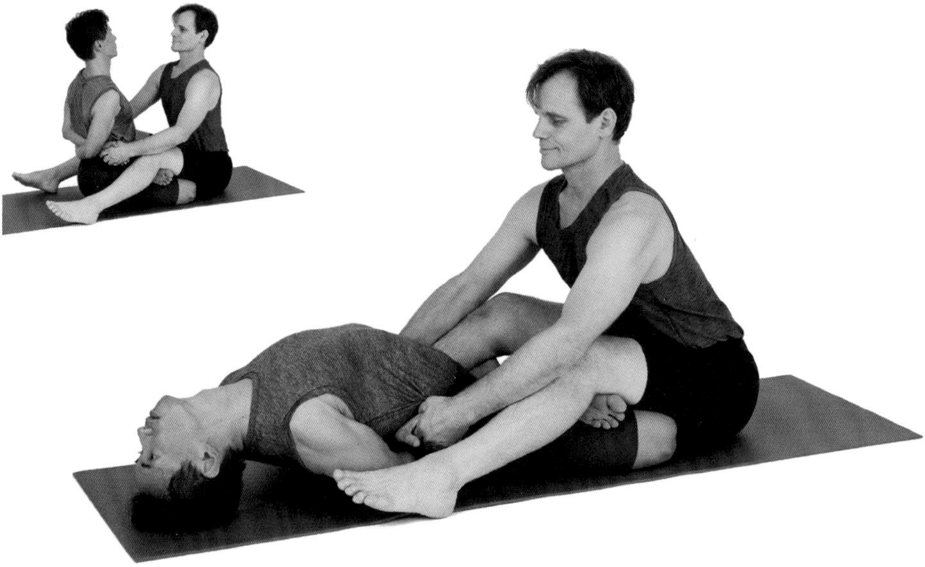

**KEY POINTS:**
This posture is performed from Baddha Padmāsana (bound lotus). If this is not possible students can use either padmāsana without the bind or sukhāsana (simple crossed-legged seat).

**ADJUSTMENT TECHNIQUES:**
Sit and place both of your own legs over the student's crossed legs and clasp the student's hands which are crossed behind the student's back. Lower the student's head to the floor 5 times. The first and last times are held for 5-10 breaths; the 2nd, 3rd and 4th repetitions are only transitions. Try to keep your own back straight throughout this assist.

**BENEFITS:**
**Muscles, Joints & Nerves:**
This posture provides a deep stretch in the shoulders, chest, belly, hips, quadriceps, and inner thighs.

**Organs & Viscera:**
Supta Vajrāsana is a variation of Baddha Padmāsana. The śloka below from Haṭha Yoga Pradīpikā highlights some of the therapeutic benefits of Baddha Padmasana, one of which is to rid the body of disease ("excrement").

The posture also is extremely beneficial for all the internal organs. The posture stretches the lungs, the diaphragm, also the area around the liver, the spleen, and all the abdominal muscles. This variation also stretches the fascia (connective tissue) for the liver, spleen, and stomach meridians.

वामोरुपरि दक्षिणं च चरं संस्थाप्य वानं तथा दक्षोरुपरि पश्चिमेन विधिना धृत्वा कराभ्यां दृधं ।
अङ्गुष्ठौ हृदये निधाय चिबुकं नासाग्रमालोकयेत् एतद् व्याधि विनाशकारि यमिनां पद्मासनं प्रोच्यते ॥ १:४४ ॥

"Bring the right foot to the root of the left thigh, then firmly place the right at the root of the left. Clasp the hands around the back and hold the big toes. Draw the chin to the chest and look at the nose tip. This padmāsana when restrained (held) has the power to cure diseases."

HAṬHA YOGA PRADĪPIKĀ 1:44

TRANSLITERATION ON PAGE 123

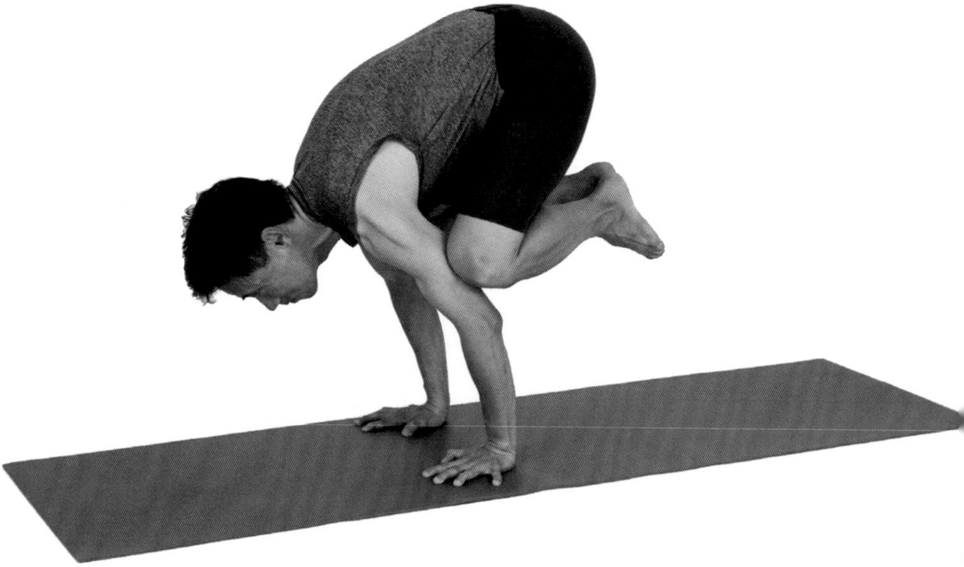

**KEY POINTS:**

Bakāsana is performed with straight arms. The knees are placed high up into armpits. The hands should be shoulder width.

If the students has wrist or shoulder problems, instead of forcing these joints, the knees should be lowered onto the mid-triceps of arms with bent elbows.

**BENEFITS:**

**Muscles, Joints & Nerves:**

Many strength postures are variations of Bakāsana, which strengthens the arms, chest, and back muscles and gives one a sense of lightness and grace while building awareness of the upper back.

Bakāsana has curative effects for those with carpal tunnel syndrome, weak arms and shoulders. Weakness in the upper back is a major factor in the misalignment of a vertbrae (sublixation) in the spinal column.

An additional benefit to strengthening the upper back is the toning of the Kūrma Naḍi situated between the shoulder blades. Patañjali author of the Yoga Sūtras states ... "Kūrma nāḍyām sthairyam" - "the Kūrma Naḍi bring stability," this applies to the mind and body.

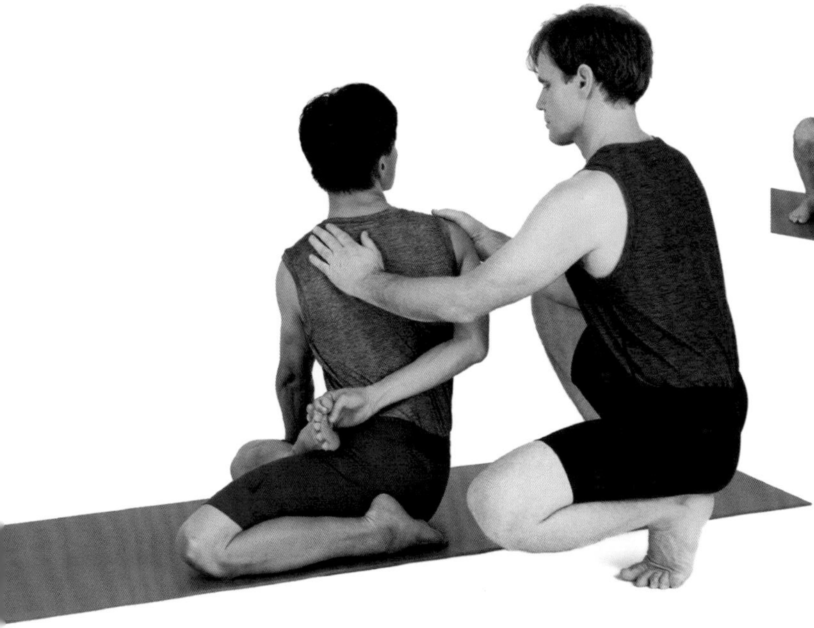

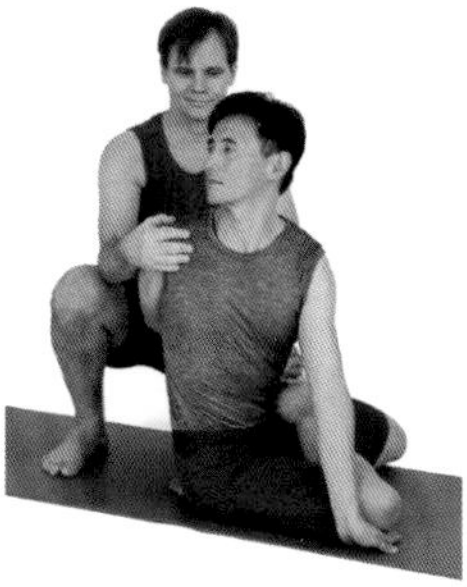

**KEY POINTS:**
This is the first of the spinal twists in the Intermediate Series. The hips should be evenly placed and the knees evenly spread from the midline of the body. The palm of the hand should be firmly placed under the thigh close to the knee.

**VARIATIONS:**
The posture can be performed without the half lotus position, by placing the bound foot under the thigh.

Students often find this posture, or a variation of it, easier to perform than the Marīcyāsana C and D and provides a good alternative to those postures if needed.

**ADJUSTMENT TECHNIQUES:**
Placing the body behind the student's back, put one hand on the student's shoulder and the other hand on the student's shoulder blade. Evenly twist the student around his/her spine.

**BENEFITS:**

**Muscles, Joints & Nerves:**
This posture tones the stomach and back muscles. It balances the internal/external obliques muscles (rib to hip muscles), the transverse abdominals, and erector spinae group (large back extension muscles). The twisting action coupled with the bound half lotus and arm placements targets the lower ribs and thereby facilitates the correct functioning of the diaphragm. This also helps to maintain the health and vitality of the spinal column.

**Organs & Viscera:**
The posture's arm placement lengthens all the fascia (connective tissue) surrounding the meridian lines of the heart, pericardium, lung, large and small intestines. The abdominal twisting action optimizes circulation in the torso. This reenergizes all the abdominal organs, including the liver, the spleen, and the large and small intestines. It also stimulates the navel area which is the home of the digestive fire (Jaṭhara Agni).

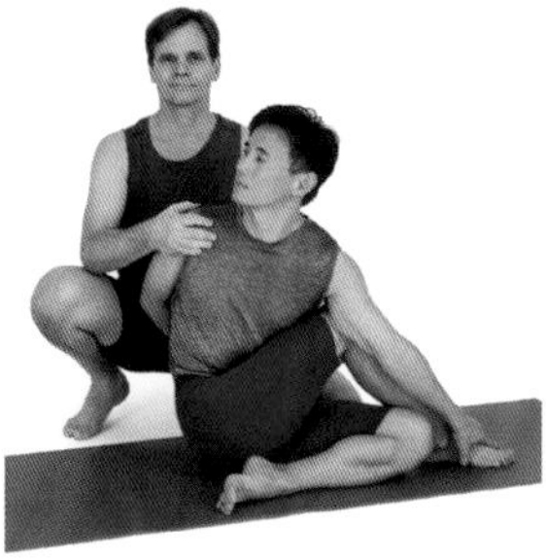

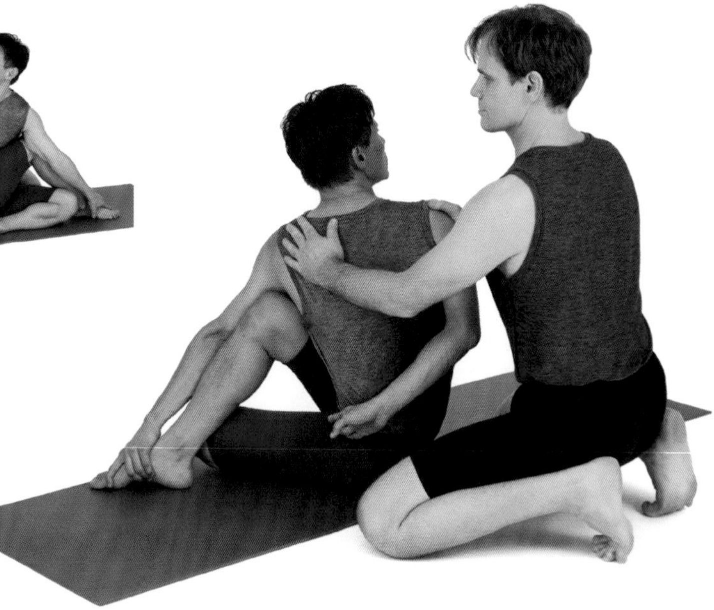

**KEY POINTS:**
Both hips should be on or close to the ground. The arm binding the front foot is stretched from the inside wrist through inner elbow and to the collarbone. The back hand holds the inner thigh.

**ADJUSTMENT TECHNIQUES:**
Place the body behind the back of the student. Hold the student around the front shoulder and back shoulder blade, and then twist the shoulders evenly around the spine.

**BENEFITS:**

**Muscles, Joints & Nerves:**
The posture provides a deep stretch in the hips. The twisting motion isolates, strengthens, and respaces the lumbar vertebrae. The whole spine receives a deep twist and the back muscles are rebalanced.

**Organs & Viscera:**
Swātmārāma, the author of the śloka below, states this posture stimulates four areas: the belly, the Khanda plexus (deep navel centre), the Kuṇḍalini (spinal energy), and the "moon" (the soft palate in the roof of the mouth). The full version, called Paripūrṇa Matsyendrāsana places the foot that is beside the hip into the half lotus position, which intensifies the pose. This posture is also beneficial for digestion and lung function.

मत्स्येन्द्रपीठां जठरप्रदीप्तं प्रचण्डरुग्मण्डलखण्डनास्त्रम् ।
अभ्यास्तः कुण्डलिनीबोधं चन्द्रस्थिरत्वं च ददाति पुम्साम् ॥ १:२७ ॥

Matsyendrapīṭhām jaṭharapradīptam pracaṇḍaruṅgmaṇḍalakhaṇḍanāstram |
abhyāsataḥ kuṇḍalinīprabodham candra sthiratvam ca dadāti pumsām || 1:27 ||

"This asana makes the belly shine and is the weapon to break open the Khañḍa circle (abdominal energetic center). Constant practice awakens the kundalini energy (spinal energy) and makes the moon (back of throat) steady." HAṬHA YOGA PRADĪPIKĀ 1:27

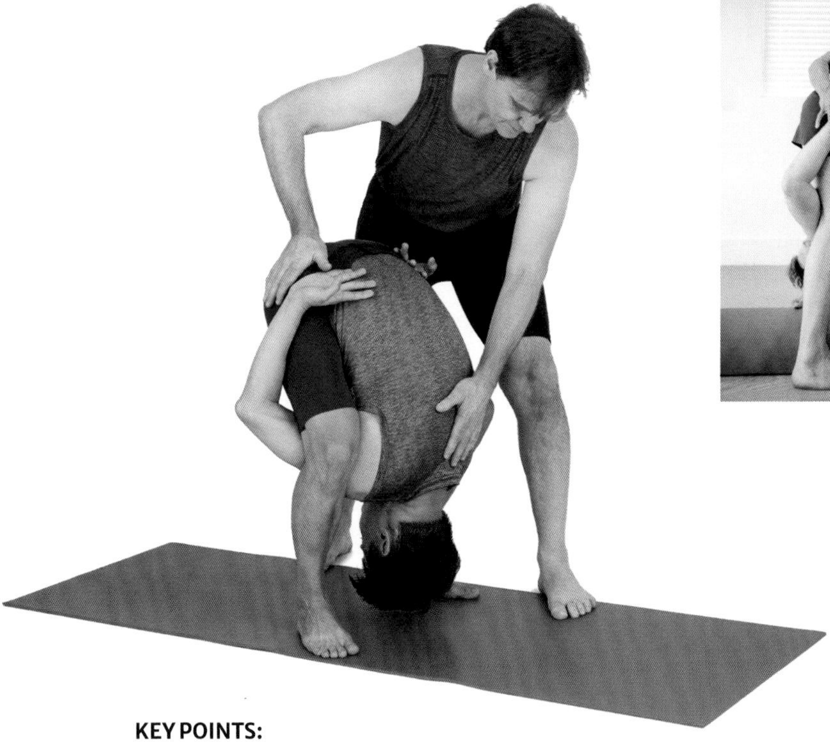

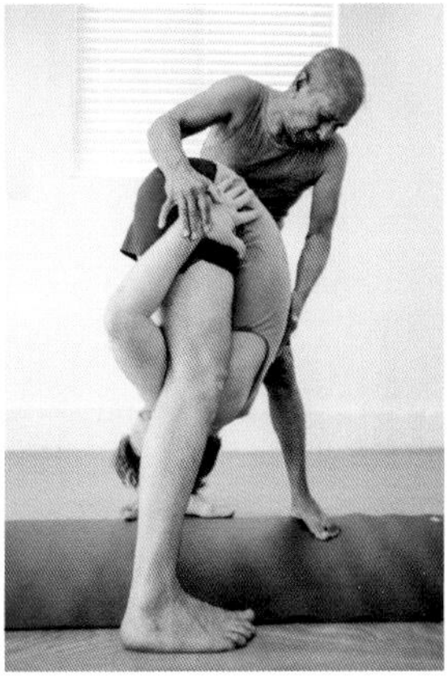

**KEY POINTS:**
Titibhāsana has three distinct sections after jumping into the posture:

1. Binding the hands behind the back (like Supta Kūrmāsana) with the feet spread apart.
2. Walking with bound hands.
3. Binding the fingers over the front of the ankles with the feet close together around bent legs. A strap can be used if the hands do not bind.

**ADJUSTMENT TECHNIQUES:**
Stand to the side of the student to help with balance if needed. The balance when the hands are around the ankles (part 3) is particularly difficult to learn; thus, a supporting hand placed on the student's hips or the back of the pelvis will steady the student.

**BENEFITS:**

**Muscles, Joints & Nerves:**
The posture fully stretches and tones the back of the legs, sacrum, and pelvic muscles. It also isolates, strengthens, and prepares the upper back for more difficult balance postures.

**Organs & Viscera:**
The posture refines one's sense of balance and challenges the vestibular system (inner ear area) for those who suffer from balance problems or dizziness. The posture relieves tension and helps clarify the nervous systems of the upper neck (cranial), base of neck and upper back (brachial), and the lower spine (lumbar) nerve plexus areas. The abdominal and reproductive organs are invigorated and the whole body feels energized from the inverse and bound stretch.

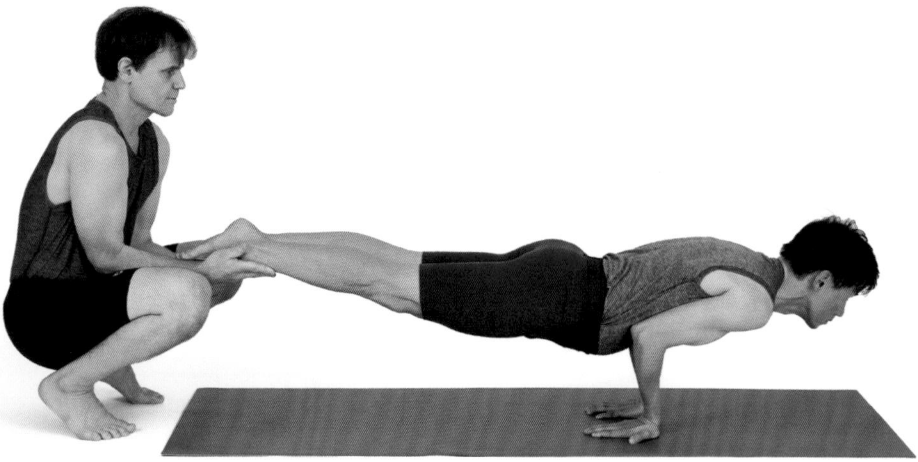

**KEY POINTS:**

The ideal shape for the posture from chin to toes is Śalabhāsana (locust posture) and is performed with straight legs. With the fingers close together, the hands are inverted and the elbows are placed close to the navel. Students must be steady over both hands.

Small variations in the leg, hand, and elbow placement can increase the accessibility of this difficult balance. If there is wrist pain, then prepare the wrists by stretching them and not taking the full weight of the body on the hands. Placing the elbows slightly apart can help in balancing. For women, an elevated leg position can be helpful. The goal is to be comfortable so one can hold the posture to secure the therapeutic benefits.

**ADJUSTMENT TECHNIQUES:**

Stand or kneel behind the student and clasp the tops of the student's feet. As the student moves the torso forward, pull the student's feet backward and up to counter balance.

**BENEFITS:**

**Muscles, Joints & Nerves:**

The posture strengthens and integrates the whole of the back of the body. Achieving the balance requires tremendous upper back strength and persistence, a benefit unto itself.

**Organs & Viscera:**

This ancient posture has been helping students for thousands of years. The pressure applied to the navel area compresses all abdominal organs and the accompanying tissue to perfect circulation in the area. This posture secures the digestive fire, the belly-centered energy for health and meditation.

हरति सकलोगानाशुगुल्मोदरादीनभिभवति च दोषानासनं श्रीमयूरम् ।
बहु कदशनभुक्तं भस्म कुर्यादशेषं जनयति जठराग्निं जारयेत्कालकूटम् ॥ १:३२ ॥

Harati sakalogānāśugulmodarādīnabhibhavati ca doṣānāsanam śrīmayūram |
bahu kadaśanabhuktam bhasma kuryādaśeṣam janayati jaṭharāgnim jārayetkālakūṭam || 1:32 ||

"This (āsana) takes (away) all diseases particularly chronic enlargement of the spleen and enlargement of the stomach. It makes the belly shine clarifying the Dośa (our Ayurvedic constitution). This great Mayūram turns to ashes the bad or remaining food (i.e. constipation), destroys the deadly poison Hālāhala, and secures the digestive fire." HAṬHA YOGA PRADĪPIKĀ 1:32

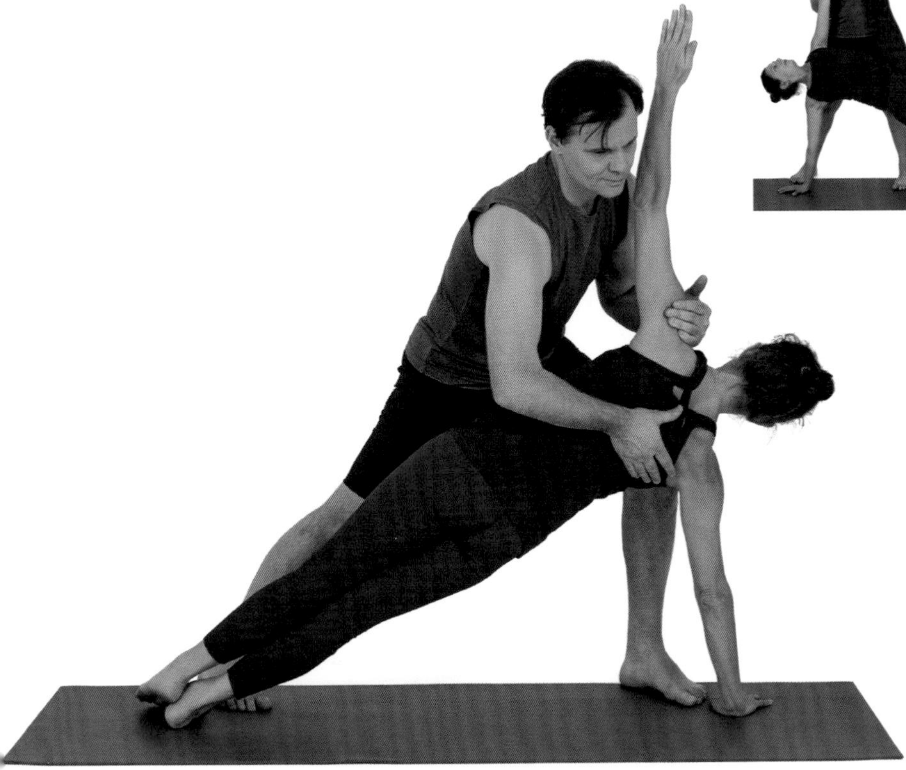

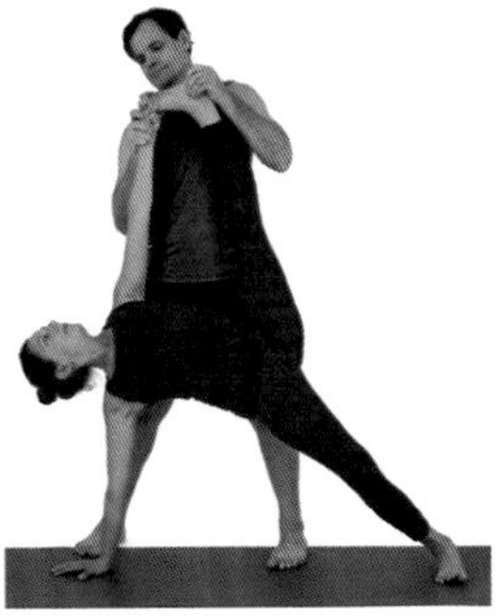

**KEY POINTS:**
This posture has two steps: a side balance with feet together; and then a side balance holding the big toe above the shoulder. Both require straight legs and straight arms. The final part is gazing toward the foot.

**ADJUSTMENT TECHNIQUES:**
Stand to the side of the student. Support the student with your hand on his/her shoulder. Use your other hand to massage the lower side of the student's back muscles from the base to neck area.

Stand on the back side of the student and support the student by helping bring the student's foot and hand together.

**BENEFITS:**
**Muscles, Joints & Nerves:**
The posture builds strength and integrates the side, back, and shoulder muscles. Additionally the posture fully works and develops the strength of the wrist and hands. This posture strengthens all the arm and leg muscles, stabilizes the shoulder and shoulder blade placement, supporting the correct chest, neck and shoulder alignment.

**Organs & Viscera:**
This is another challenging posture to balance in and is a good challenge for the vestibular (inner ear) system.

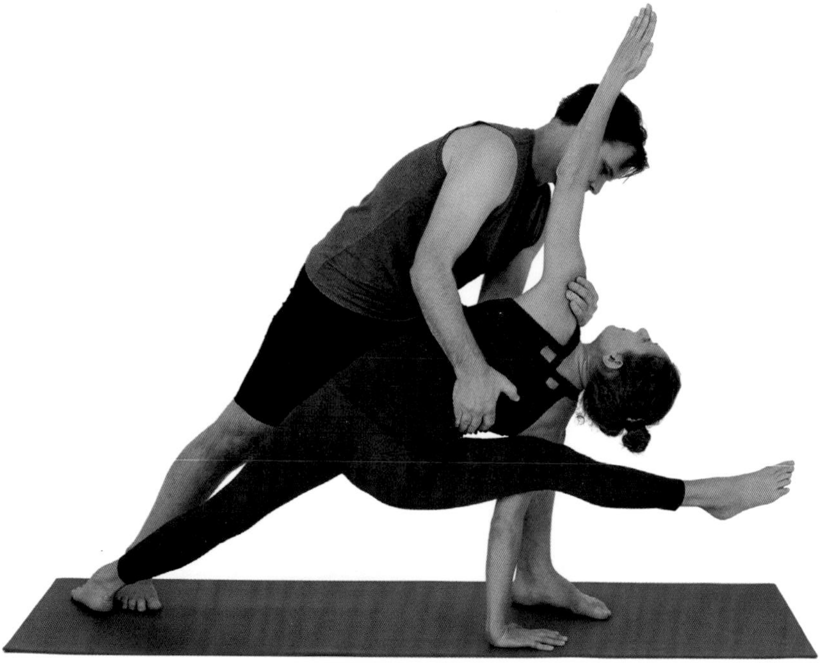

**KEY POINTS:**
Vaśiṣṭhāsana is ideally performed with straight legs and arms. The knee of the stretched leg is tucked tightly against the upper back and shoulder blade then the gaze rests up to the fingertips.

**ADJUSTMENT TECHNIQUES:**
Standing on the front side of the student, reach around the student's back and support the waist. Use your other hand to support and hold the student's shoulder.

**BENEFITS:**

**Muscles, Joints & Nerves:**
Viśvamitrāsana encourages the correct functioning of the thoracic spine and has curative effects for spinal issues like Scoliosis (4 or more vertebrae twisted in a row), Kyphosis and Lordosis (excessive hunching and inward curvature of the spine). The debilitating effects of a vertebral subluxation (misalignment of one or more vertebrae) is dramatically decreased as the muscle tone is established to draw the spine back into alignment.

**Organs & Viscera:**
Both Vaśiṣṭhāsana and Viśvamitrāsana integrate and stabilize all the vertabrae. This is tremendously helpful for the long term health of the spine. Both these postures are named after ancient Indian sages and help develop the qualities of these sages in those who meditate in them.

Yoga therapy is not just about flexibility and alignment. The advanced series poses that Manju has chosen develop dynamic strength and vitality in the body.

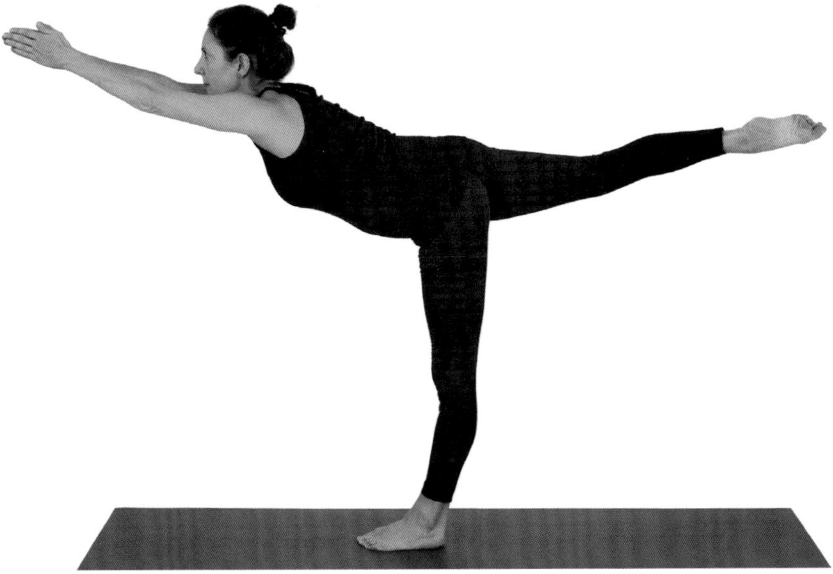

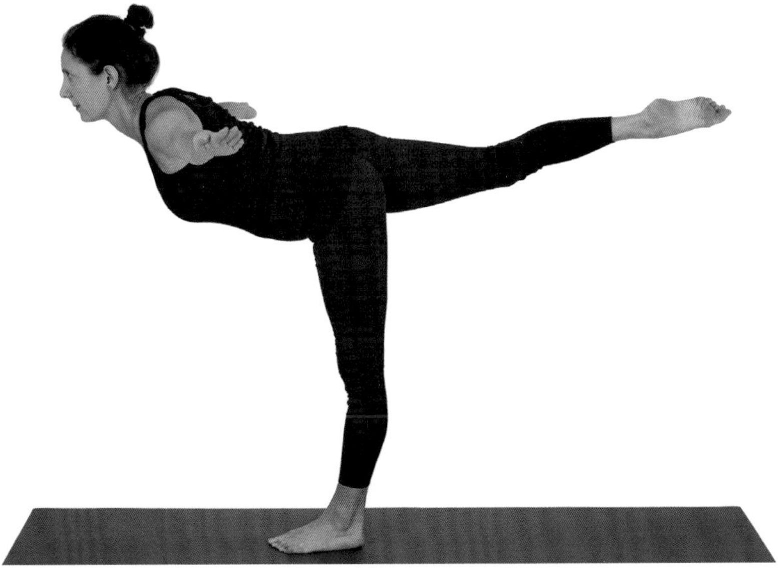

**KEY POINTS:**
The student's body from the arms to the toes of the raised leg should be parallel to the floor. The arms and legs are either straight out from the shoulders or with the palms joined and arms next to the head.

**BENEFITS:**
**Muscles Joints & Nerves:**
One develops a sense of the whole line of the body from toe to head. The posture challenges the vestibular system and strengthens the body. It especially tones the sacral and upper back musculature. Changing the arm positions strenthens the muscles closer to the spine.

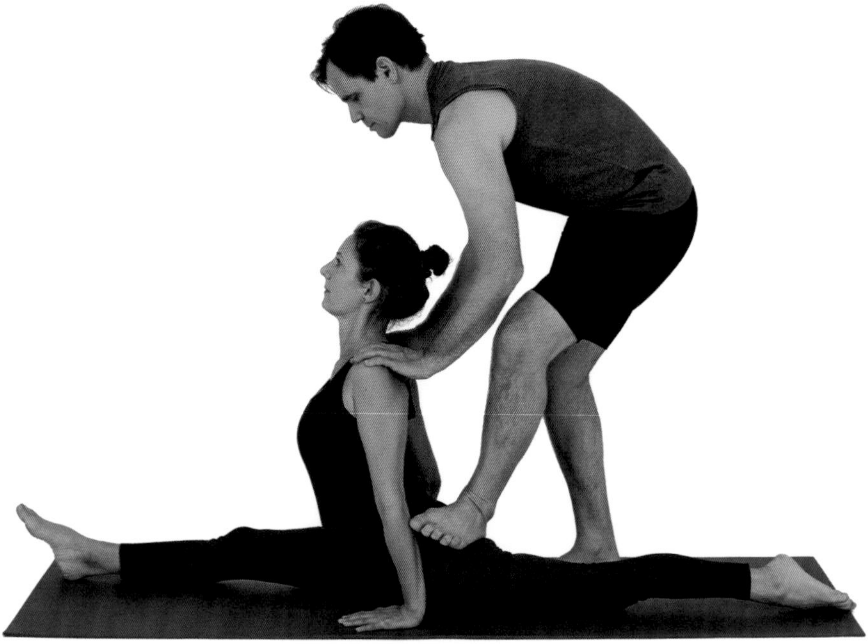

**KEY POINTS:**
This posture should be performed with the spine upright, like in Daṇḍasana, and straight legs. The back leg should be rotated so the upper thigh and knee are on the floor.

**ADJUSTMENT TECHNIQUES:**
The adjustment facilitates bringing the back hip towards the floor. Hold the student's shoulders to balance the student and then use the pressure of your foot to ease the student's hip down. If needed cushions, or blankets can be used to raise the hips off the ground and relieve pressure and give access to the posture.

**BENEFITS:**

**Muscles Joints & Nerves:**
This posture creates equal and opposite pressure through the right and left sides of the pelvis and hips. It fully opens the hip area in flexion and creates a deep relaxation through the hip flexors (psoas), buttocks and stomach muscles. The posture restores the natural movement between the pelvis and sacrum and removes impingements in the sciatic (lower spine through buttock into the back leg) and femoral (lower spine through front pelvis into the inner leg) nerve pathways to improve leg muscle functionality.

**Organs & Viscera:**
The posture improves circulation to the organs in the pelvis and the abdominal cavity. Because it relaxes the diaphragm, chest muscles, and back rib muscles breathing is improved.

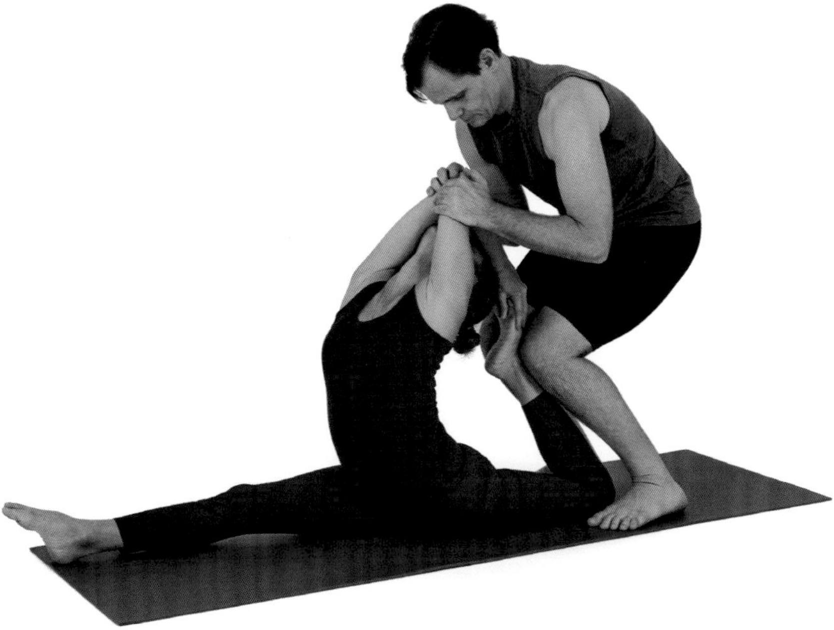

**KEY POINTS:**
The posture, which is named after a saw, is a variation on Hanumanāsana. The front leg should be stretched directly forward, and the back hip should be fully down. The back knee is then bent, and one grabs hold the back foot and rests the head on sole of the foot.

**MODIFICATIONS:**
If the hamstring group of the front thigh is not fully developed, blankets and bolsters/blocks can be used to raise the hips off the floor and relieve the pressure.

**ADJUSTMENT TECHNIQUES:**
Stand behind the student and secure the student's foot between your own knees and thighs. After the student reaches the hands over the head, bring the student's hands to the foot, and draw the foot and head close together.

**BENEFITS:**
**Muscles, Joints & Nerves:**
The posture has the same benefits as Hanumanāsana. However, it additionally stretches the whole abdominal cavity, the chest and throat muscles. Because of the intense chest and back muscle stretch the body is prepared for prāṇāyāma.

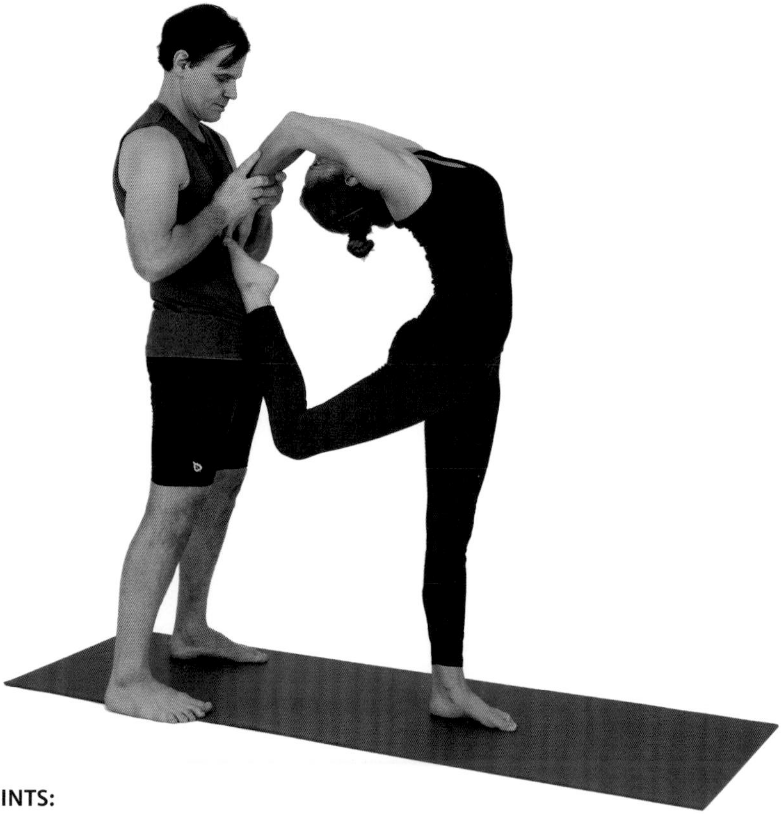

**KEY POINTS:**
This posture requires drawing the back foot up to meet the hands in line with the shoulders. Ideally, the foot is clasped by the hands above the head.

**ADJUSTMENT TECHNIQUES:**
Stand behind the student's bent leg and allow the foot to rest on your torso. Then pull the student's hands back to the foot.

As an alternative, stand to the side of the student and help lift the student's knee and elbow into position while the student maintains the grip on the foot.

**BENEFITS:**

**Muscles, Joints & Nerves:**
It takes tremendous upper back strength and flexibility to perform this posture. It benefits the entire spine by freeing up the shoulders, shoulder blades, and ribs.

**Organs & Viscera:**
The posture provides a deep squeeze to the kidney and adrenal gland areas. It also invigorates the whole nervous system.

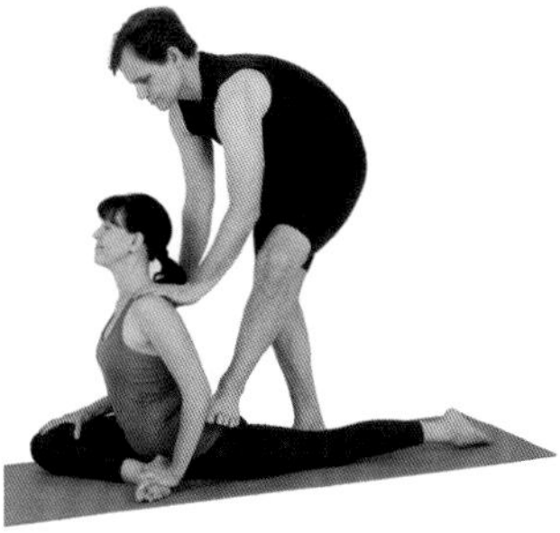

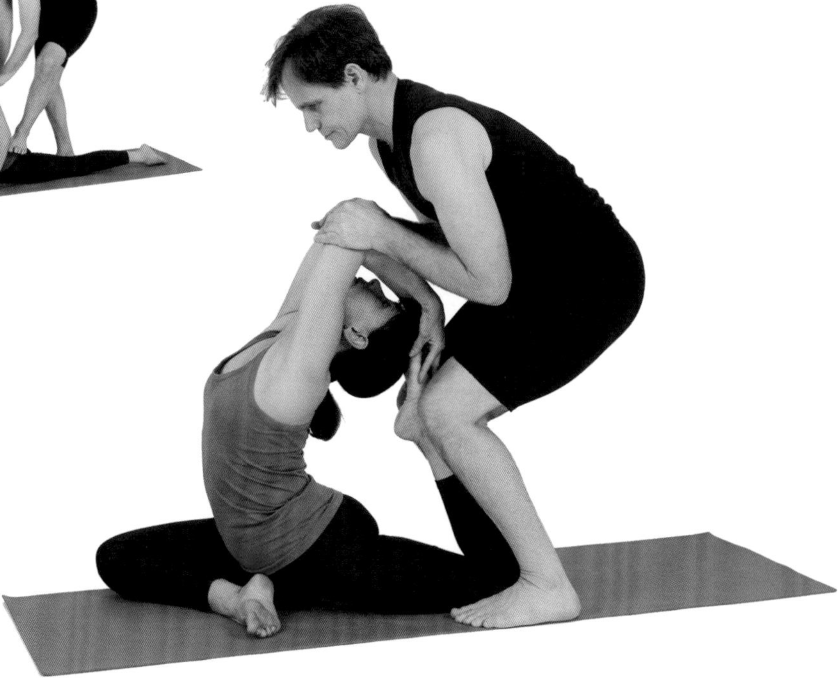

**KEY POINTS:**
Commonly referred to as Pigeon (Kapo) posture. The back thigh and front folded leg should be fully grounded. The torso twists inward, while the back thigh remains grounded as you bend backwards. The student reaches over the head to clasp the foot, ideally with two hands.

**ADJUSTMENT TECHNIQUES:**
Standing at the rear of the student secure their back knee between your feet and knees. Your knees hold the students body steady. As the student arches clasp their hands (or forearms) and bring them to the foot. Once the student is comfortable draw the elbows together.

**BENEFITS:**

**Muscles, Joints & Nerves:**
A deep stretch is felt through the whole spine. The sacroiliac joint, the thoracic spine and rib attachments are rebalanced. The sacral and lumbar nerve plexuses, are toned. The sciatic pathway through the pelvis, including piriformus muscle is released. The femoral nerve pathways for the front thigh musculature is rebalanced.

All the front abdominal muscles, including psoas major and minor (hip flexors), obliques, rectus abdominus, and the diaphragm are stretched and rebalanced. The back spinal erector muscles are fully engaged and strengthened, a tremendous help for maintaining a healthy vertebral column.

**Organs & Viscera:**
The whole abdominal cavity and the digestive organs are respaced and toned while the twisting nature of the posture targets the colon. Any problems with Duodenum and reflux can be cured through this posture.

"Surya Namaskara – A yoga asana connected with breath movement. How you use the breath to move on to the posture. This is the best way to get movement back in the body."

"In the old times, they would do "a yoga prayer" – everything was done in Sankrit – the surya namaskara were all a prayer. Everyone is doing it at the same time. It becomes like a spiritual dance."

Manju Jois

**Nava vinyāsa**
**Ekam** - in, arms up
**Dwe** - ex, hands to feet, head down
**Trīṇi** - in, look up, straight arms
**Catvāri** - ex, caturaṅga daṇḍāsana
**Pañca** - in, ūrdhva mukha śvānāsana
**Ṣat** - ex, adho mukha śvānāsana
**Nabhi dṛṣṭi**
**Daśa dīrgha recaka pūraka**
**Sapta** - in, jump feet to hands, look up
**Aṣṭau** - ex, head down
**Nava** - in, arms up
**Samasthitiḥ** - ex, hands to sides

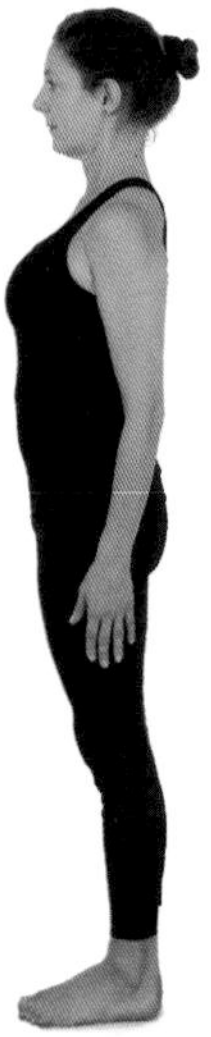

**Samasthitiḥ**

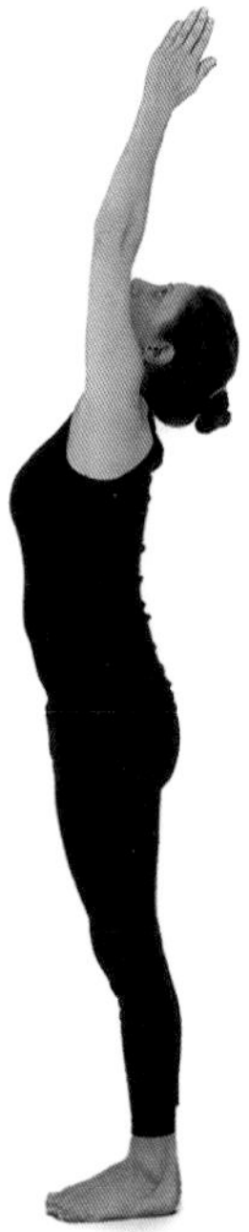

**Ekam**

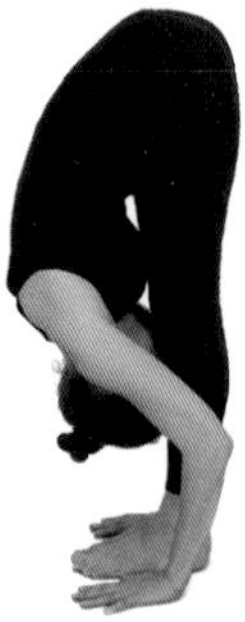

**Dwe**

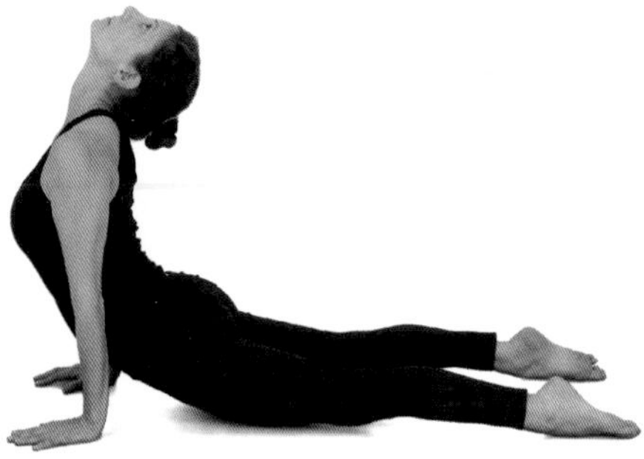

**Pañca**

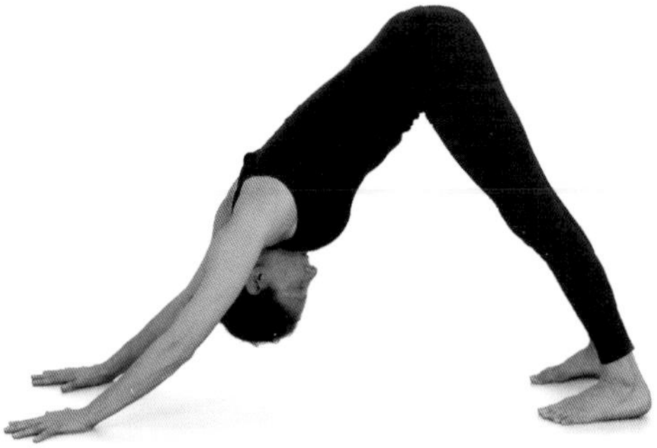

**Ṣat**

Nāda Yoga, the yoga of sound, is a huge part of Manju's approach. He often plays traditional Indian music in his class and is known for his beautiful chanting.

The following pages give the text (script) for the vinyasas in Sanskṛt for Primary and Intermediate series. Additional text gives explanation/cues/directions as needed.

"Nāda tanumani śam" The combination of mind, body & sounds brings peace.

– Traditional Indian Verse

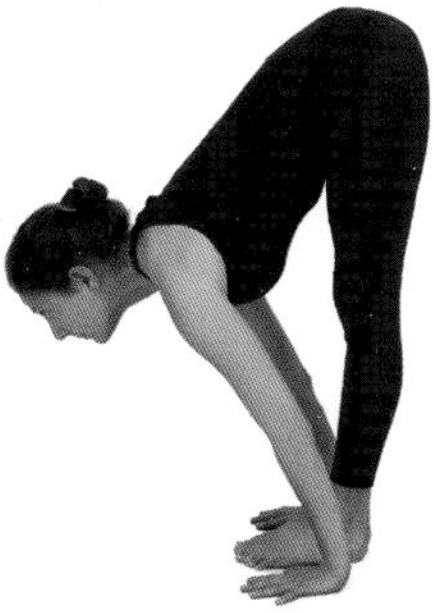

**Trīṇi**

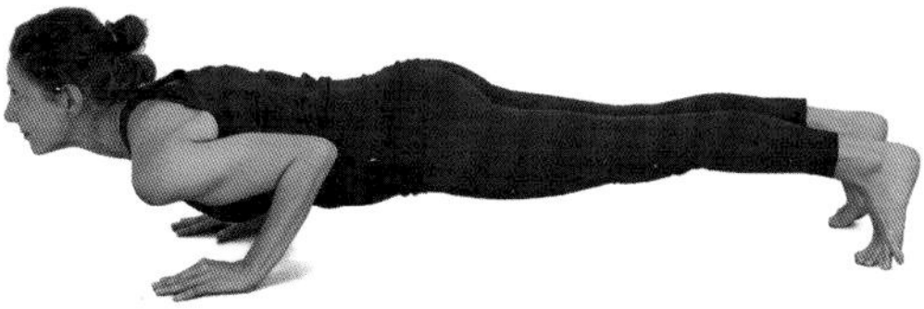

**Catvāri**

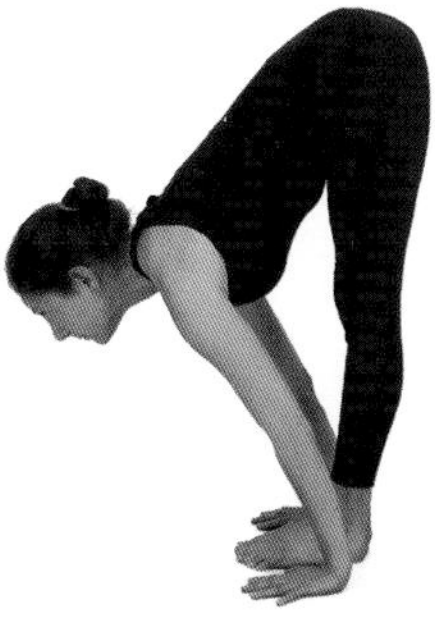

**Sapta**

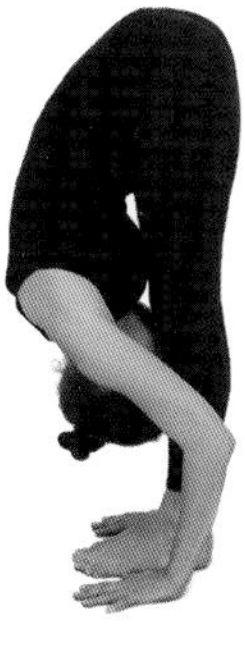

**Aṣṭau**

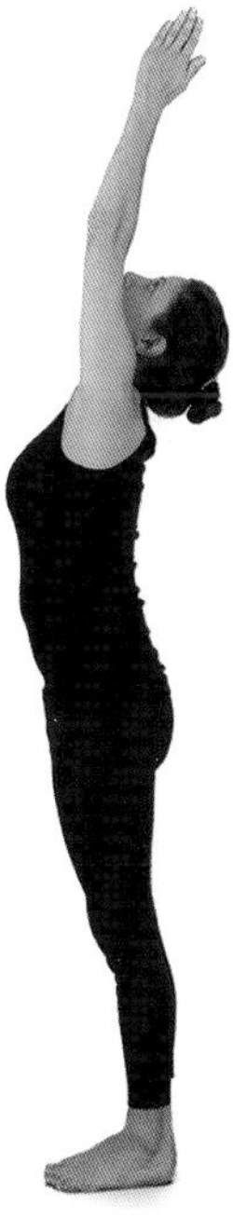

**Nava**

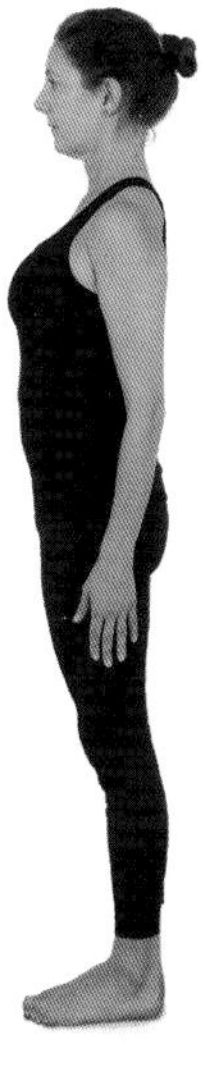

**Samasthitiḥ**

**Saptadaśa vinyāsa**
**Ekam** - in, arms up (Utkaṭāsana position)
**Dwe** - ex, hands to feet, head down
**Trīṇi** - in, look up, straight arms
**Catvāri** - ex, caturaṅga daṇḍāsana
**Pañca** - in, ūrdhva mukha śvānāsana
**Ṣat** - ex, adho mukha śvānāsana
**Sapta** - in, right foot forward (Vīrabhadrāsana position)
**Aṣṭau** - ex, caturaṅga daṇḍāsana
**Nava** - in, ūrdhva mukha śvānāsana
**Daśa** - ex, adho mukha śvānāsana
**Ekādaśa** - in, left foot forward (Vīrabhadrāsana position)
**Dvādaśa** - ex, caturaṅga daṇḍāsana
**Trayodaśa** - in, ūrdhva mukha śvānāsana
**Caturdaśa** - ex, adho mukha śvānāsana
**Nabhi dṛṣṭi**
**Daśa dīrgha recaka pūraka**
**Pañcadaśa** - in, jump feet to hands, look up
**Ṣodaśa** - ex, head down
**Saptadaśa** - in, arms up (Utkaṭāsana position)
**Samasthitiḥ** - ex, hands to sides

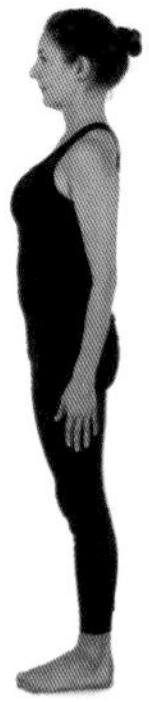

**Samasthitiḥ**

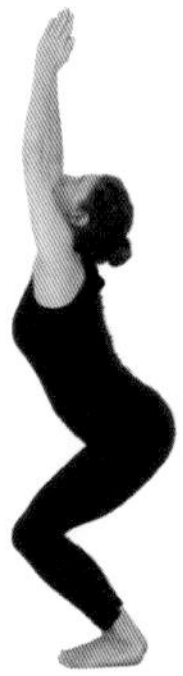

**Ekam**

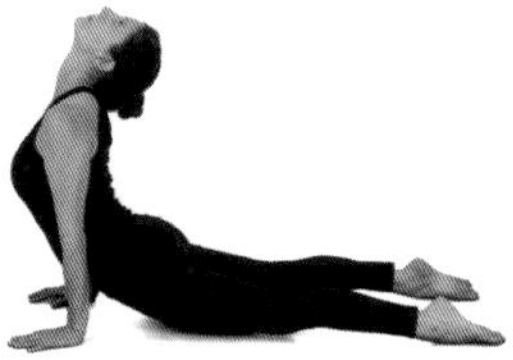

**Pañca**

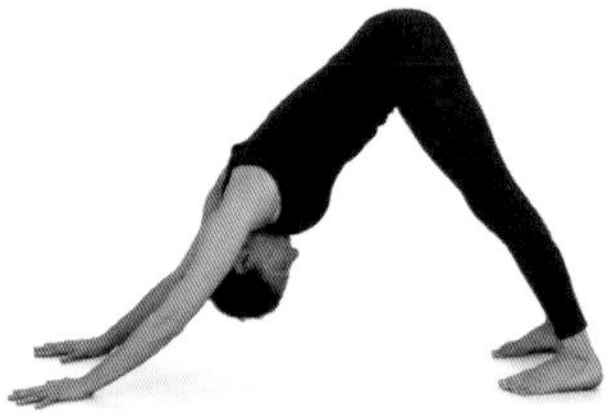

**Ṣat**

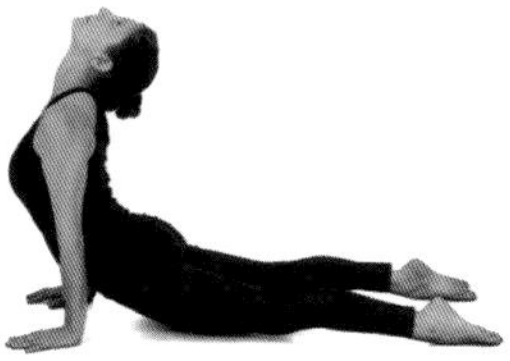

**Nava**

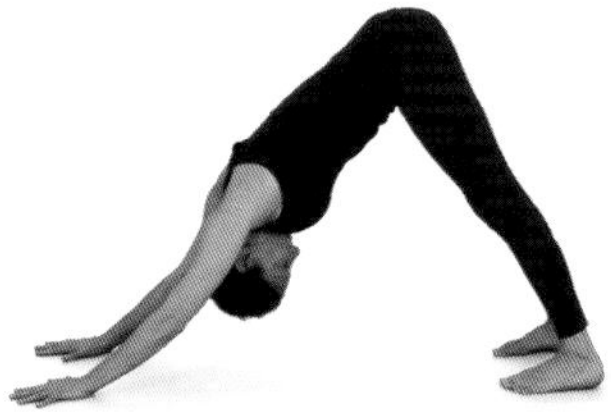

**Daśa**

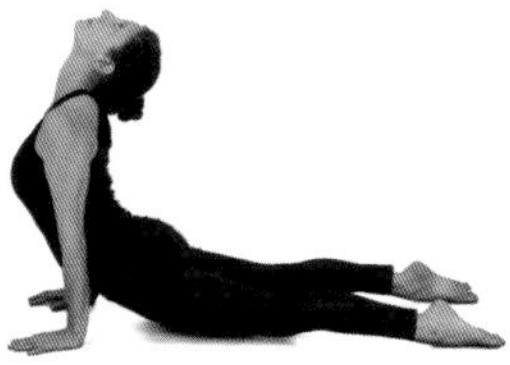

**Trayodaśa**

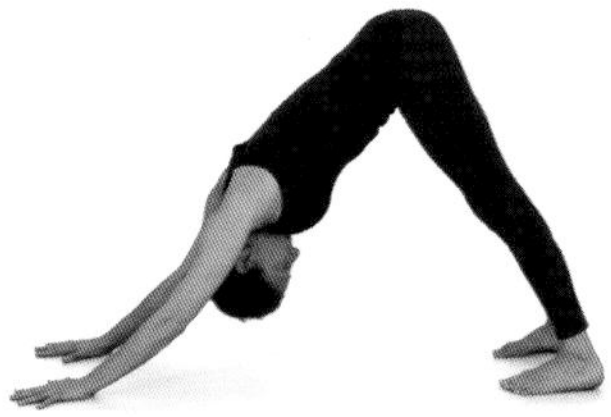

**Caturdaśa**

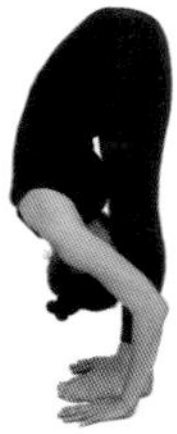

Dwe

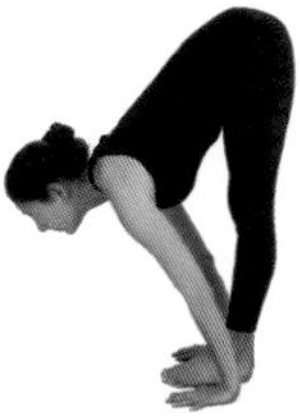

Trīṇi

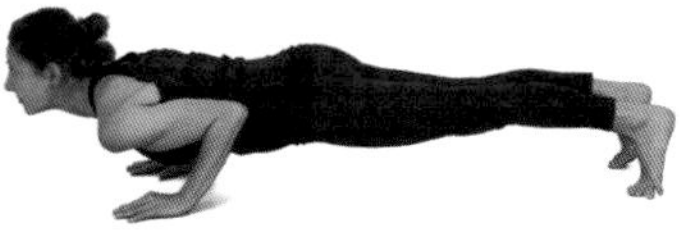

Catvāri

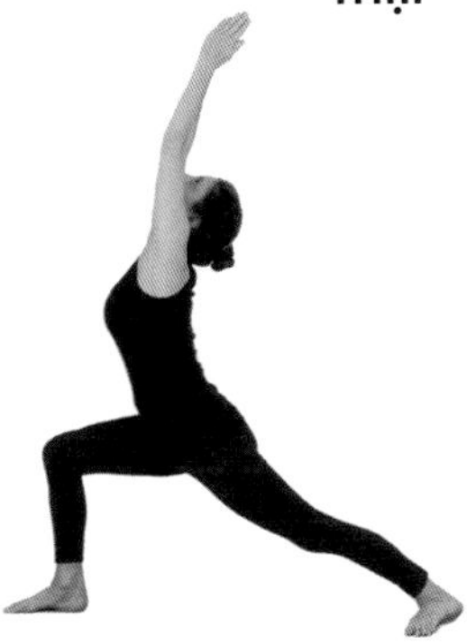

Sapta

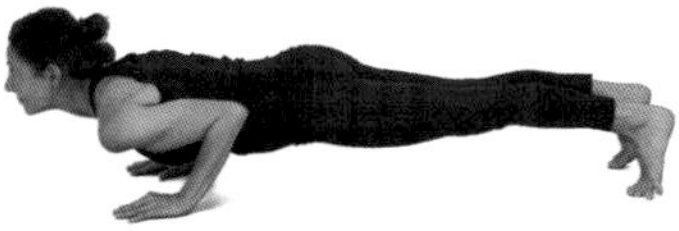

Aṣṭau

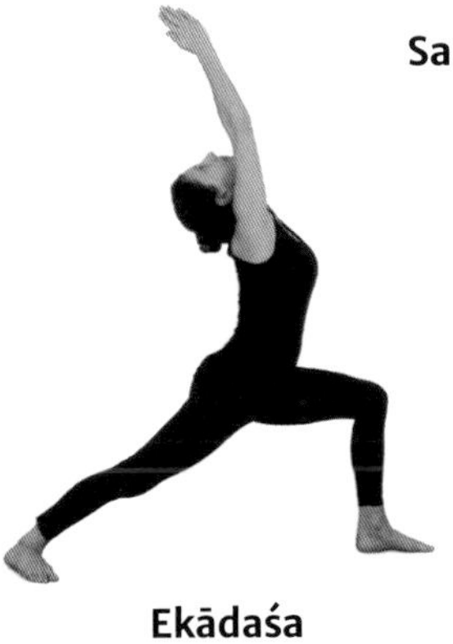

Ekādaśa

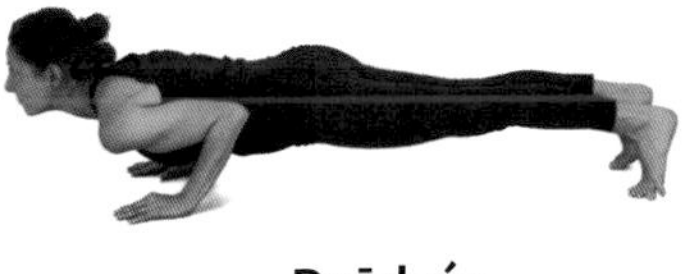

Dvādaśa

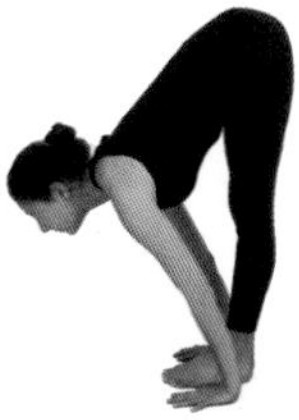

Pañcadaśa

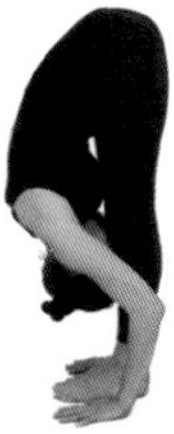

Ṣodaśa

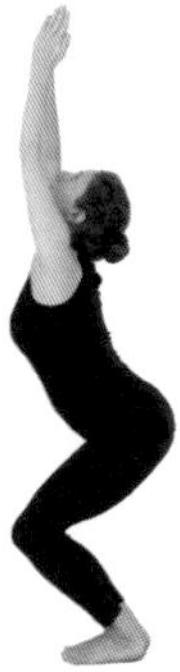

Saptadaśa

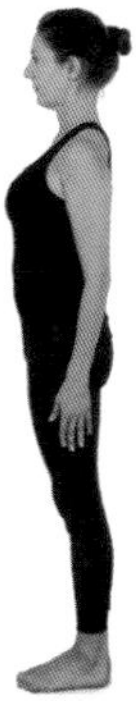

Samasthitiḥ

"The standing postures are a complete sequence. As a teacher you can see the problems in a student's body highlighted in the standing poses."

Manju Jois

## Pādāṅguṣṭhāsanam पादाङ्गुष्ठासनम्

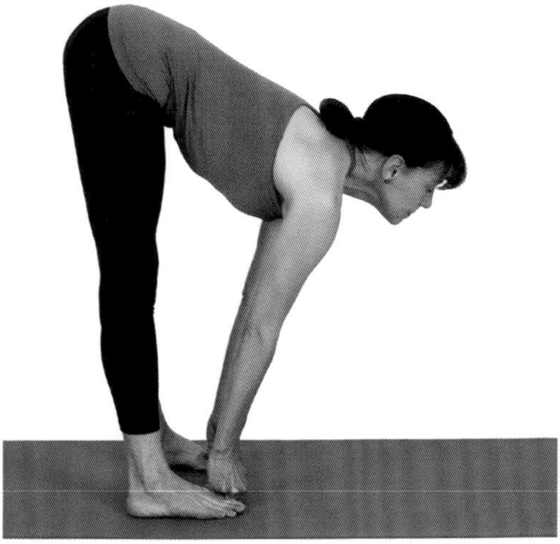

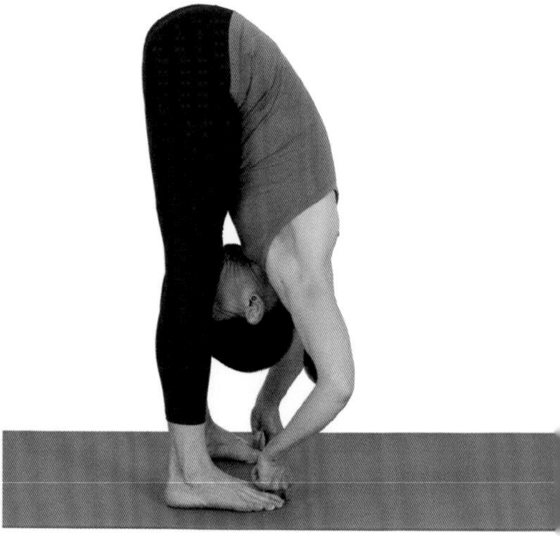

**Ekam** - hold big toes with first two fingers and thumb, in
**Dwe** - ex, take position
**Nasāgra dṛṣṭi**
**Daśa dīrgha recaka pūraka**
**Trīṇi** - in, stretch arms, head up

## Pādahastāsana पादहस्तासन

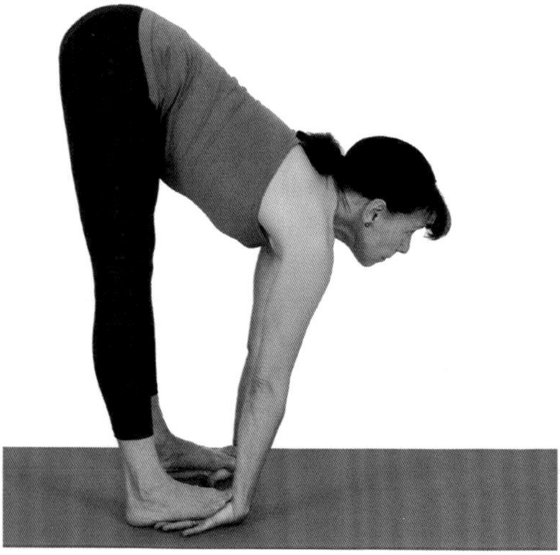

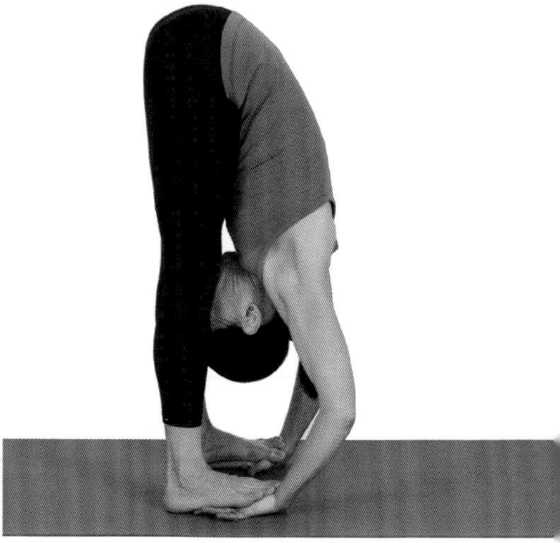

**Ekam** - place palms under feet head up, in
**Dwe** - ex, head down
**Nasāgra dṛṣṭi**
**Daśa dīrgha recaka pūraka**
**Trīṇi** - in, stretch arms, head up
**Samasthitiḥ**

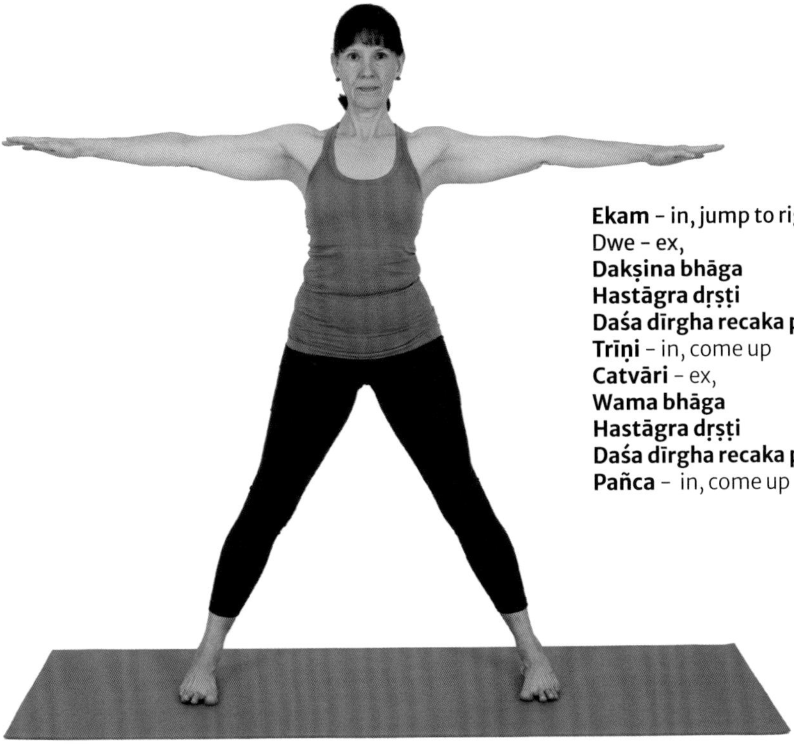

**Ekam** - in, jump to right
Dwe - ex,
**Dakṣina bhāga**
**Hastāgra dṛṣṭi**
**Daśa dīrgha recaka pūraka**
**Trīṇi** - in, come up
**Catvāri** - ex,
**Wama bhāga**
**Hastāgra dṛṣṭi**
**Daśa dīrgha recaka pūraka**
**Pañca** - in, come up

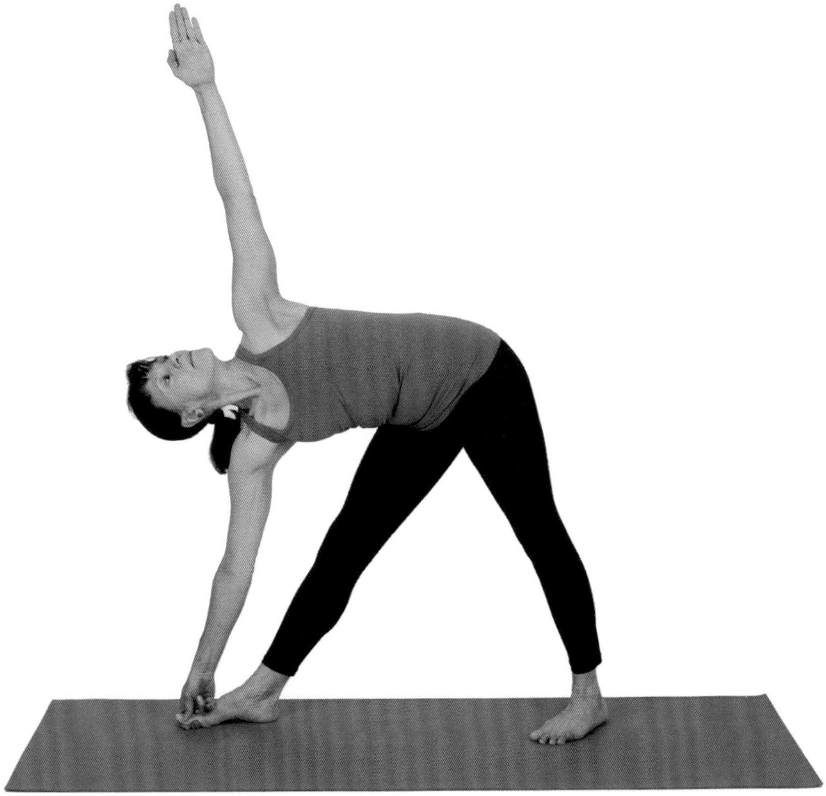

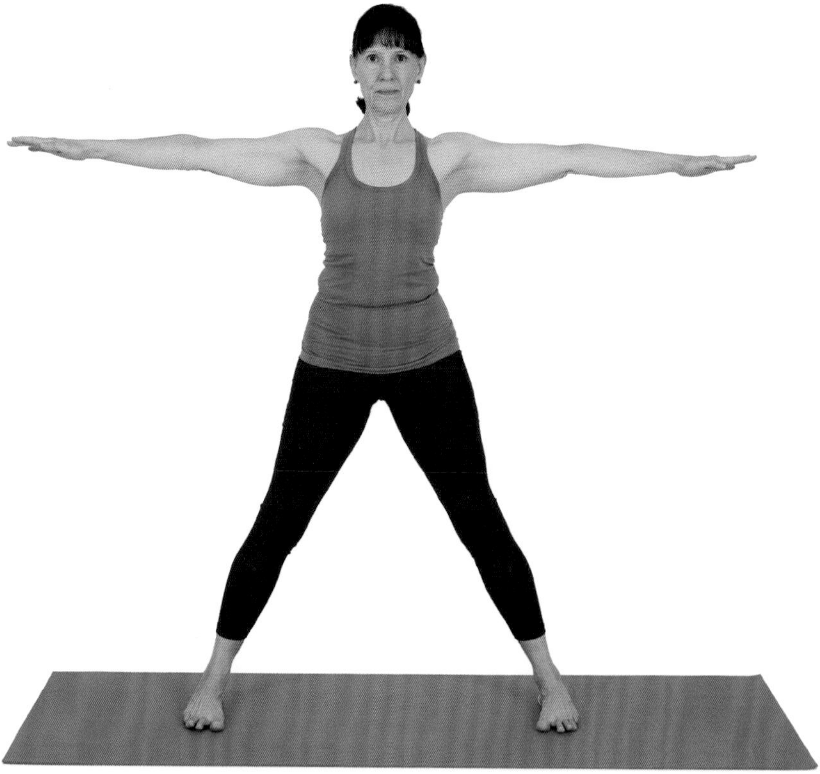

**Dwe** - ex, dakṣina bhāga
**Hastāgra dṛṣṭi**
**Daśa dīrgha recaka pūraka**
**Trīṇi** - in, come up
**Catvāri** - ex,
**Wama bhāga**
**Hastāgra dṛṣṭi**
**Daśa dīrgha recaka pūraka**
Pañca - in, come up
**Samasthitiḥ**

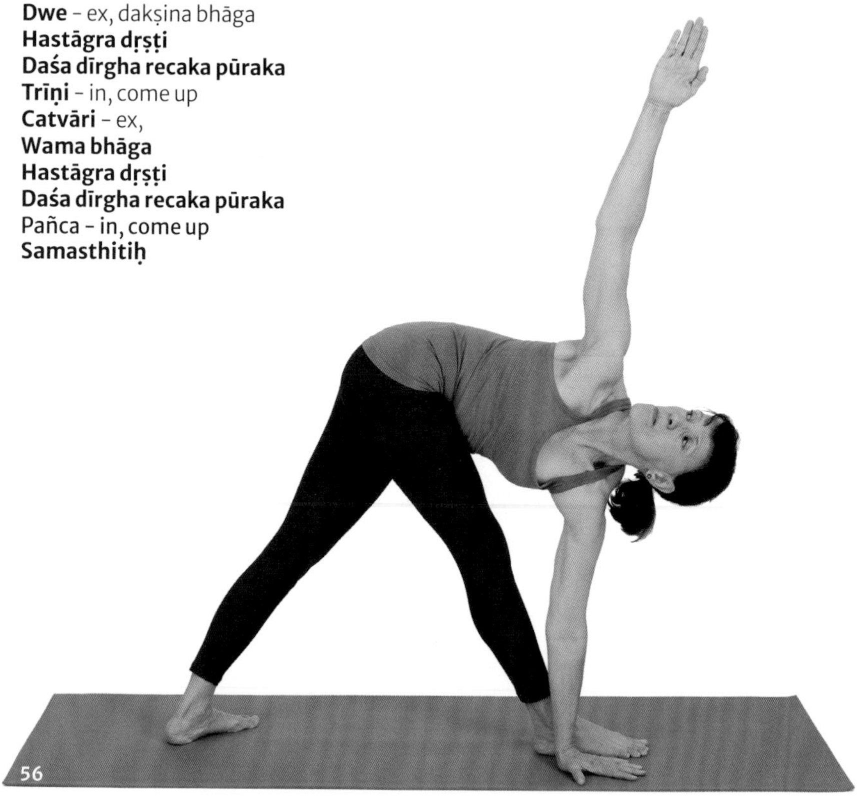

## Utthita Pārśva Koṇāsanam
## उत्थित पार्श्व कोणासनम्

**Ekam** – in, jump to right
**Dwe** – ex,
**Dakṣina bhāga**
**Hastāgra dṛṣṭi**
**Daśa dīrgha recaka pūraka**
**Trīṇi** – in, come up
**Catvāri** – ex,
**Wama bhāga**
**Hastāgra dṛṣṭi**
**Daśa dīrgha recaka pūraka**
**Pañca** – in, come up

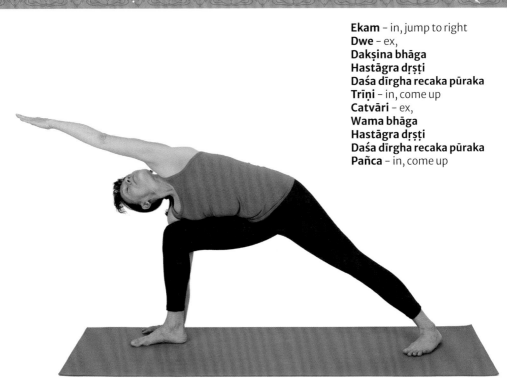

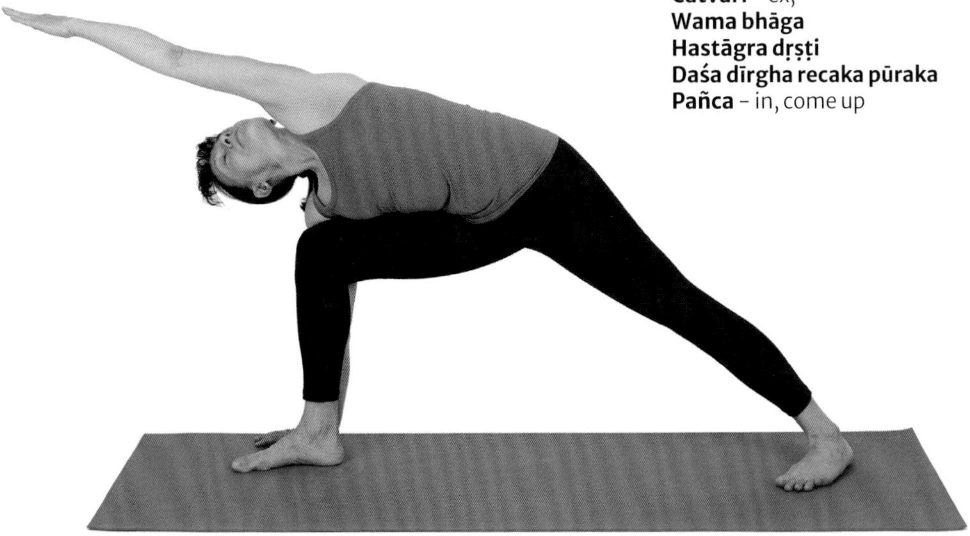

## Parivṛtta Pārśva Koṇāsanam
## परिवृत्त पार्श्व कोणासनम्

**Dwe** – ex,
**Dakṣina bhāga**
**Hastāgra dṛṣṭi**
**Daśa dīrgha recaka**
**Trīṇi** – in, come up
**Catvāri** – ex,
**Wama bhāga**
**Hastāgra dṛṣṭi**
**Daśa dīrgha recaka pūraka**
**Pañca** – in, come up
**Samasthitiḥ**

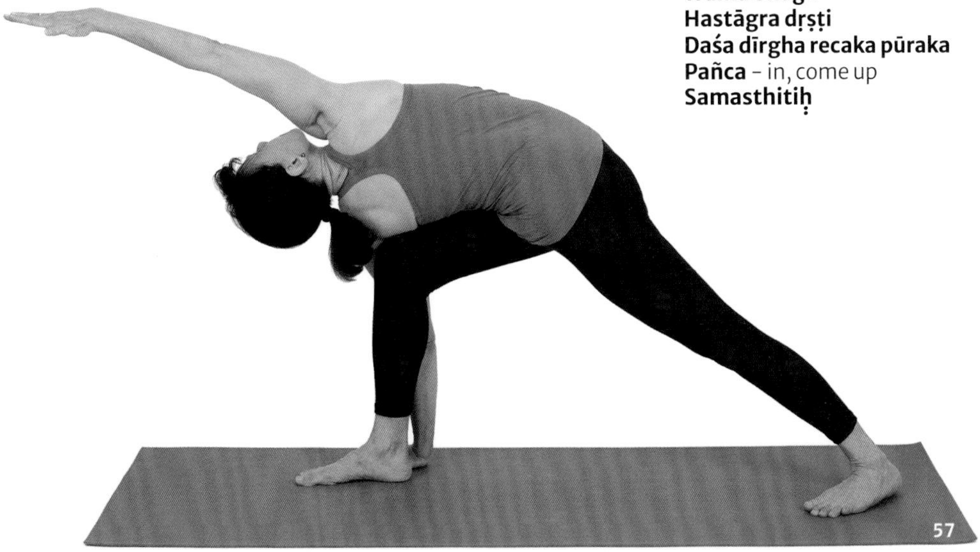

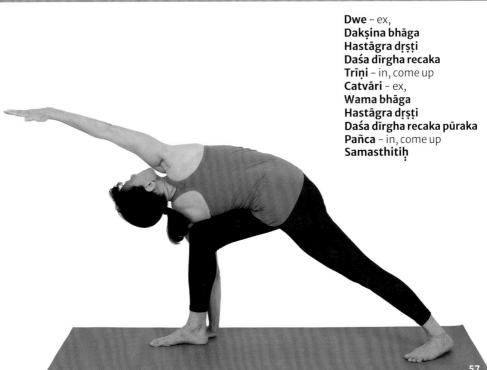

## Prathama Prasārita Pādottānāsanam प्रथम प्रसारित पादोत्तानासनम्

**Ekam** - in, jump out, hands on waist
**Dwe** - ex, forward bend hands, between legs, in
**Trīṇi** - ex, head between legs
**Nasāgra dṛṣṭi**
**Daśa dīrgha recaka pūraka**
**Catvāri** - in, straighten arms, ex
**Pañca** - in, come up

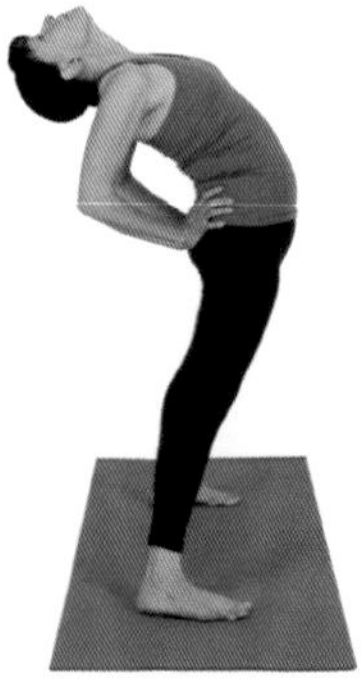

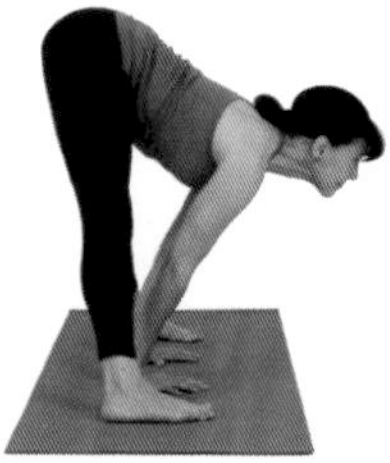

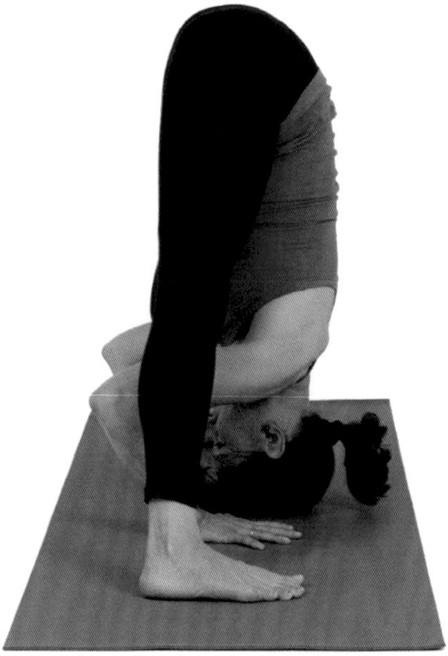

## Dwitīya Prasārita Pādottānāsanam द्वितीय प्रसारित पादोत्तानासनम्

**Ekam** - in, arms out
**Dwe** - ex, hand to waist
**Trīṇi** - in, arch the back
**Catvāri** - ex, head between legs
**Nasāgra dṛṣṭi**
**Daśa dīrgha recaka pūraka**
**Pañca** - in, come up

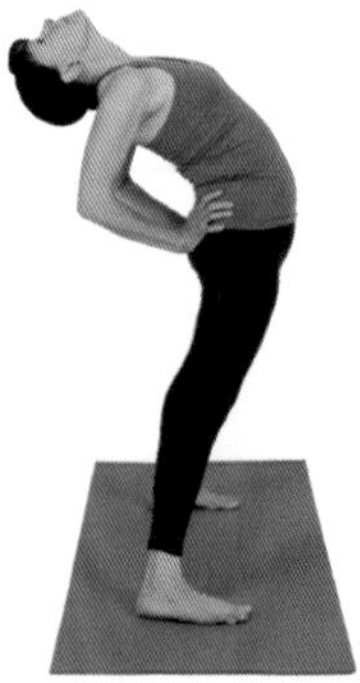

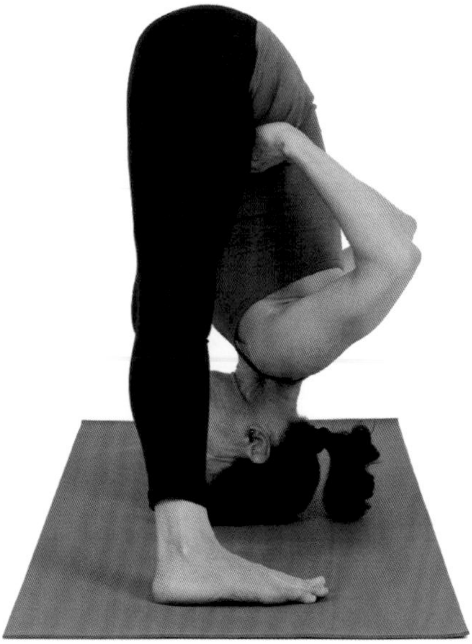

## Tṛtīya Prasārita Pādottānāsanam तृतीय प्रसारित पादोत्तानासनम्

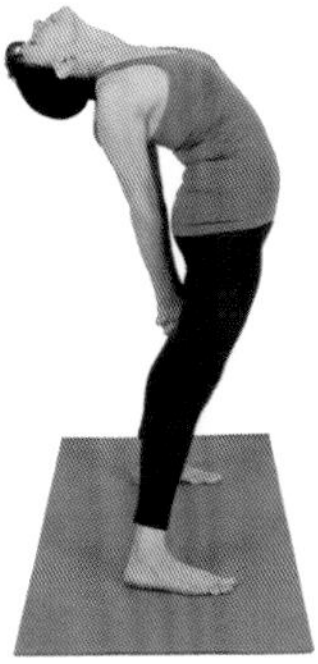

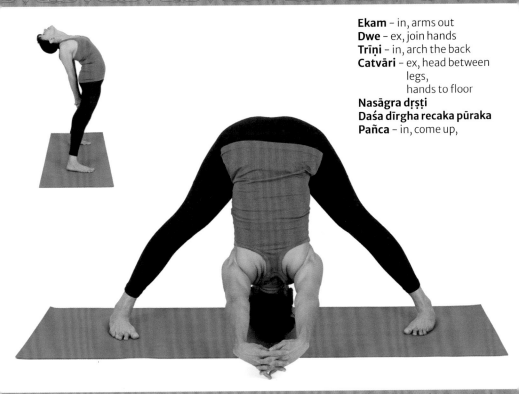

**Ekam** – in, arms out
**Dwe** – ex, join hands
**Trīṇi** – in, arch the back
**Catvāri** – ex, head between legs, hands to floor
**Nasāgra dṛṣṭi**
**Daśa dīrgha recaka pūraka**
**Pañca** – in, come up,

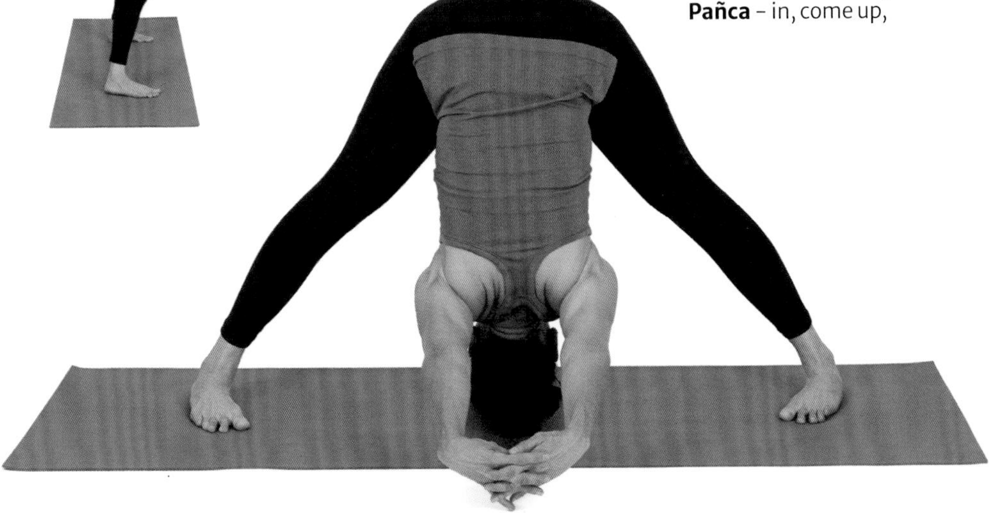

## Caturtha Prasārita Pādottānāsanam चतुर्थ प्रसारित पादोत्तानासनम्

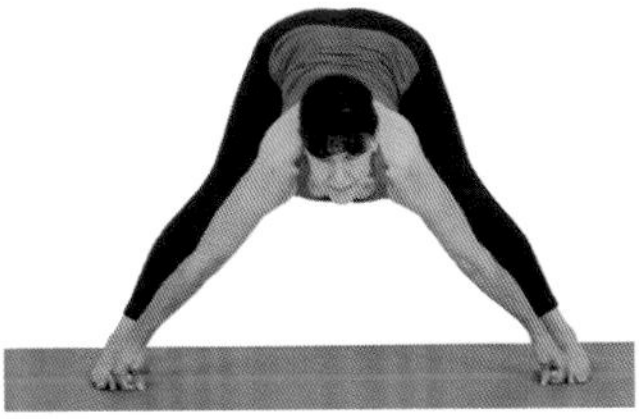

**Ekam** – in, hands on waist
**Dwe** – ex, forward bend hold big toes, in
**Trīṇi** – ex, head between legs
**Nasāgra dṛṣṭi**
**Daśa dīrgha recaka pūraka**
**Catvāri** – in, straighten arms, ex
**Pañca** – in, come up
**Samasthitiḥ**

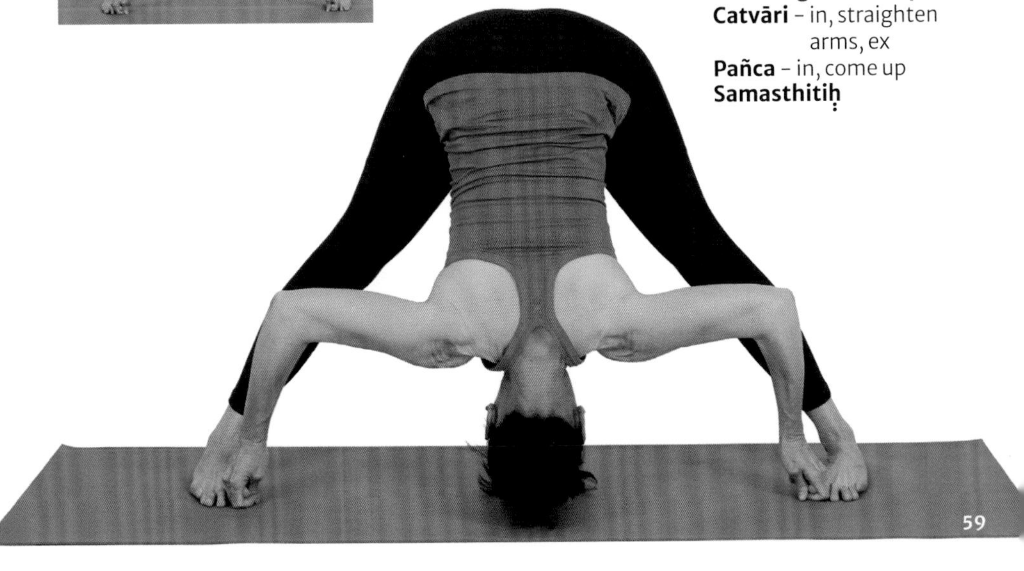

**Ekam** - in, jump to right, join palms behind back
**Dwe** - ex,
**Dakṣina bhāga**
**Nasāgra dṛṣṭi**
**Daśa dīrgha recaka pūraka**
**Trīṇi** - in, come up
**Catvāri** - ex,
**Wama bhāga**
**Dakṣina bhāga**
**Nasāgra dṛṣṭi**
**Daśa dīrgha recaka pūraka**
**Pañca** - in, come up
**Samasthitiḥ**

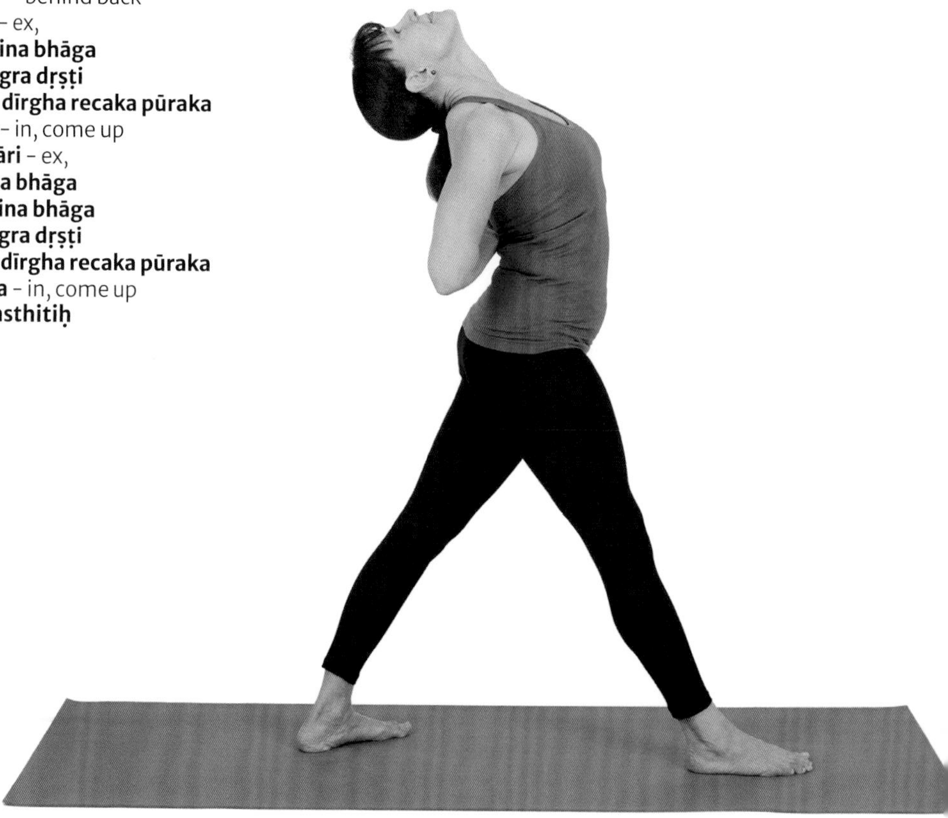

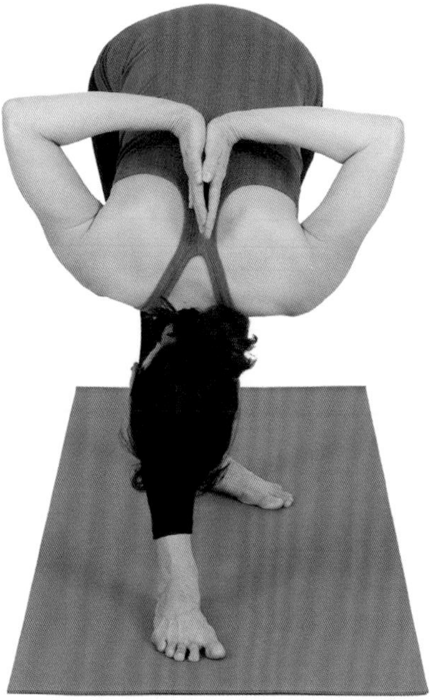

**Dakṣina bhāga**
**Ekam** - leg up hold right big toe, in
**Dwe** - ex, forward bend
**Nasāgra dṛṣṭi**
**Daśa dīrgha recaka pūraka**
**Trīṇi** - in, come up
**Catvāri** - ex, leg to side
**Pārśva dṛṣṭi**
**Daśa dīrgha recaka pūraka**
**Pañca** - in, leg to the front
**Ṣat** - ex, forward bend
**Sapta** - in, come up, hands to waist
**Nasāgra dṛṣṭi**
**Daśa dīrgha recaka pūraka**
**Samasthitiḥ**
**Utthita Hasta Pādāṅguṣṭhāsana**
**Wama bhāga**
(same as right side - Dakṣina bhāga)

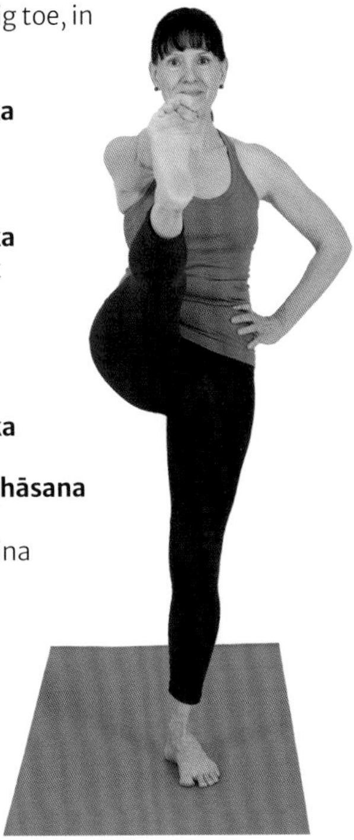

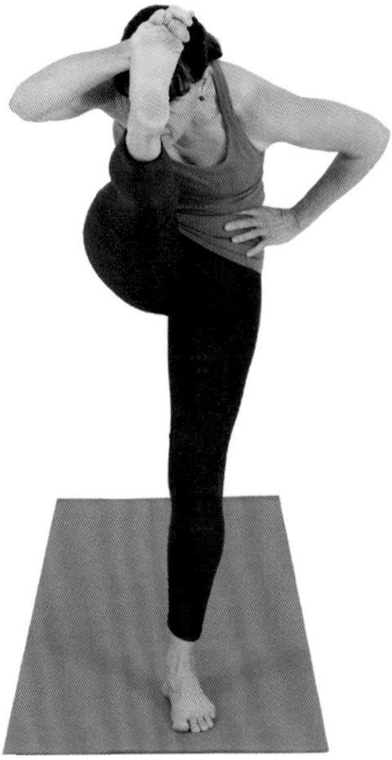

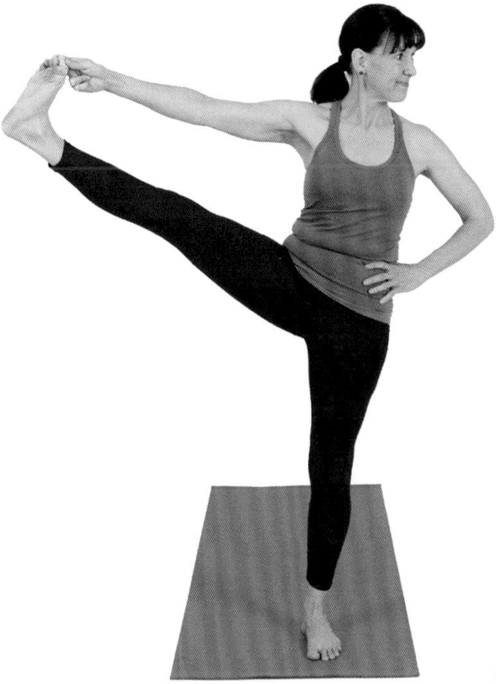

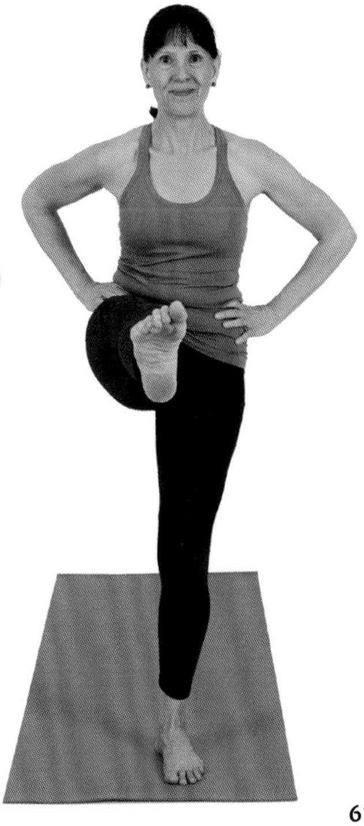

**Dakṣina bhāga**
**Ekam** - in, right foot up, bind foot
**Dwe** - ex, hand beside foot, in
**Trīṇi** - ex, forward bend
**Daśa dīrgha recaka pūraka**
**Nasāgra dṛṣṭi**
**Catvāri** - in, head up, ex
**Pañca** - in, come up
**Samasthitiḥ**
**Ardha Baddha Padmottānāsana**
**Wama bhāga**
(same as right side - Dakṣina bhāga)

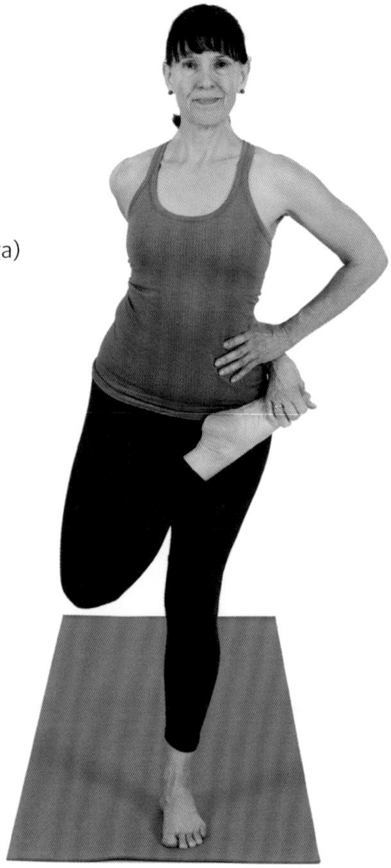

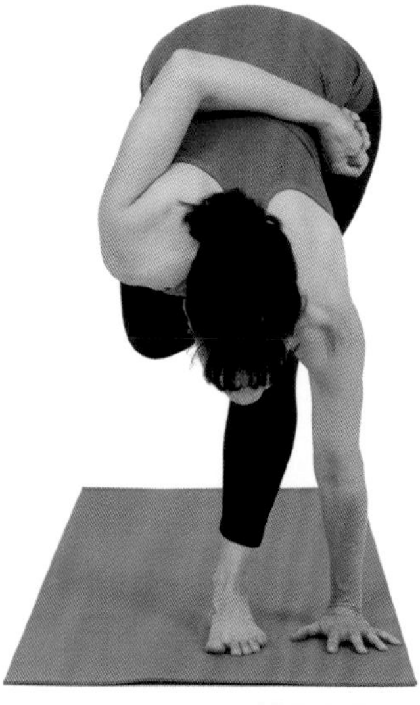

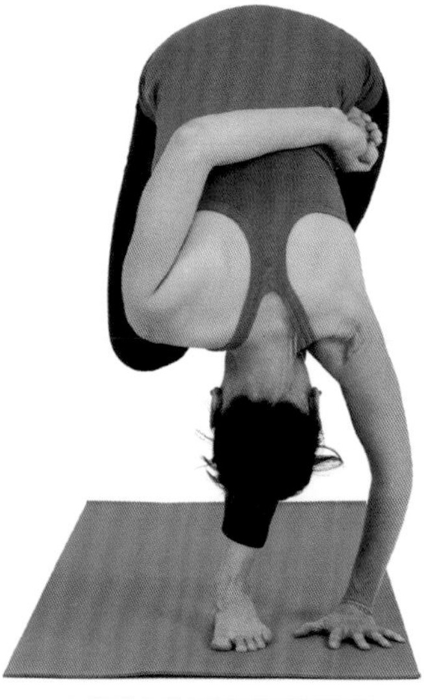

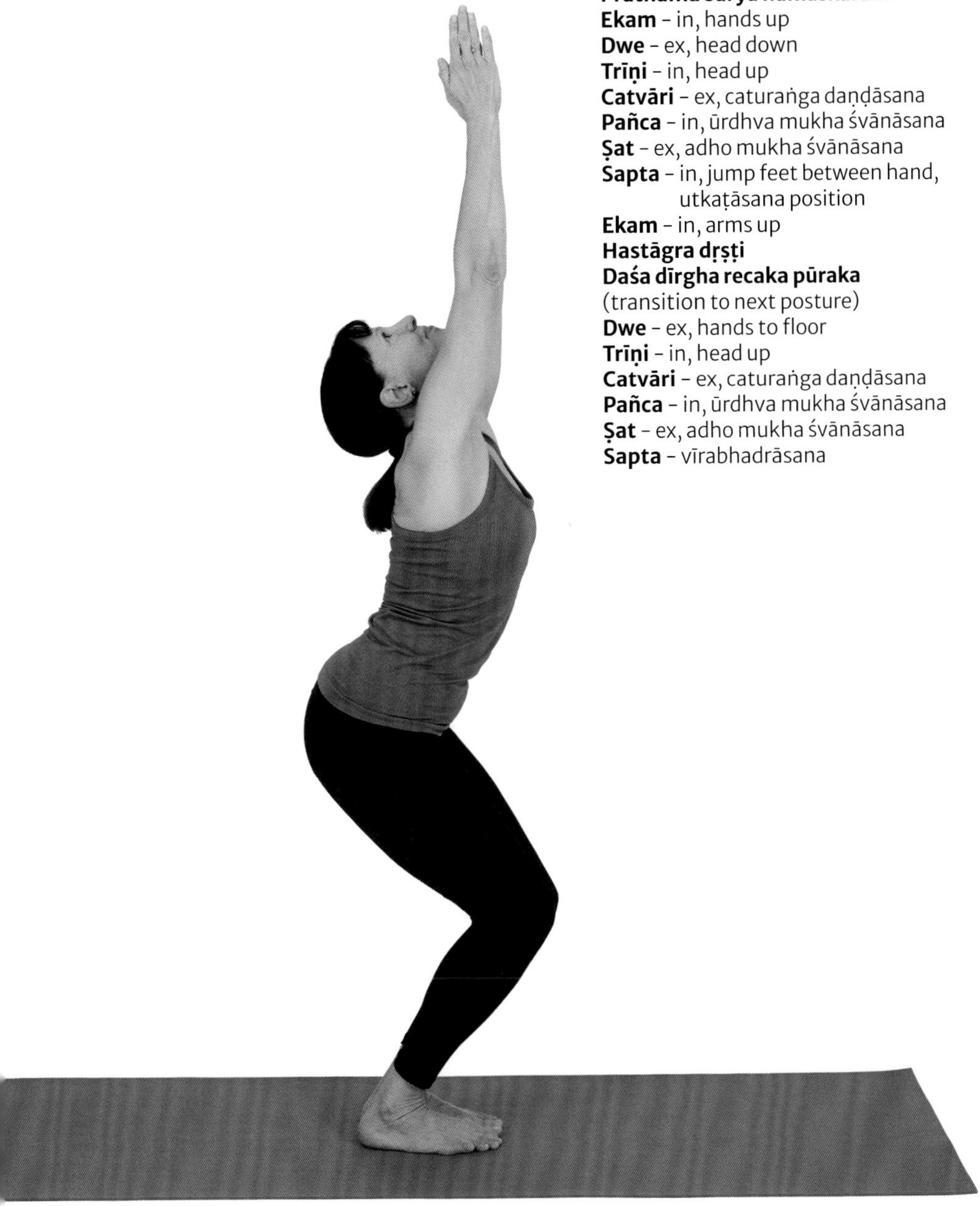

**Prathama sūrya namaskāram**
**Ekam** - in, hands up
**Dwe** - ex, head down
**Trīṇi** - in, head up
**Catvāri** - ex, caturaṅga daṇḍāsana
**Pañca** - in, ūrdhva mukha śvānāsana
**Ṣat** - ex, adho mukha śvānāsana
**Sapta** - in, jump feet between hand, utkaṭāsana position
**Ekam** - in, arms up
**Hastāgra dṛṣṭi**
**Daśa dīrgha recaka pūraka**
(transition to next posture)
**Dwe** - ex, hands to floor
**Trīṇi** - in, head up
**Catvāri** - ex, caturaṅga daṇḍāsana
**Pañca** - in, ūrdhva mukha śvānāsana
**Ṣat** - ex, adho mukha śvānāsana
**Sapta** - vīrabhadrāsana

अङ्गुष्ठाभ्यामवष्टभ्य धरां गुल्फौ च खे गतौ ।
तत्रोपरि गुदं न्यसेद्विज्ञेयमुत्कटासनम् ॥ २:२७ ॥

Anguṣṭhābhyāmavaṣṭabhya dharām gulphau cha khe gatau |
tatropari gudam nyased vijñeyamutkaṭāsanam || 2:27 ||

Rest both big toes (& feet) and ankles on the floor, then above set down the anus (deeply bending the knees). This Utkaṭāsana (fierce position) is wise yogic practice. GHERAṆḌA SAMHITA 2:27

**Ekam** - in, right foot forward
**Hastāgra dṛṣṭi**
**Daśa dīrgha recaka pūraka**
**Dwe** - turn to back
**Hastāgra Dṛṣṭi**
**Daśa dīrgha recaka pūraka**
**Trīṇi** - arms out, left knee bent, facing back
**Pārśva dṛṣṭi,** (left)
**Daśa dīrgha recaka pūraka**
**Catvāri** - second side
**Pārśva dṛṣṭi** (right)
**Daśa dīrgha recaka pūraka**
(Utpluthiḥ)
(transition to next posture)
**Pañca** - ex, caturaṅga daṇḍāsana
**Ṣat** - in, ūrdhva mukha śvānāsana
**Sapta** - ex, adho mukha śvānāsana
**Aṣṭau** - in, daṇḍāsana

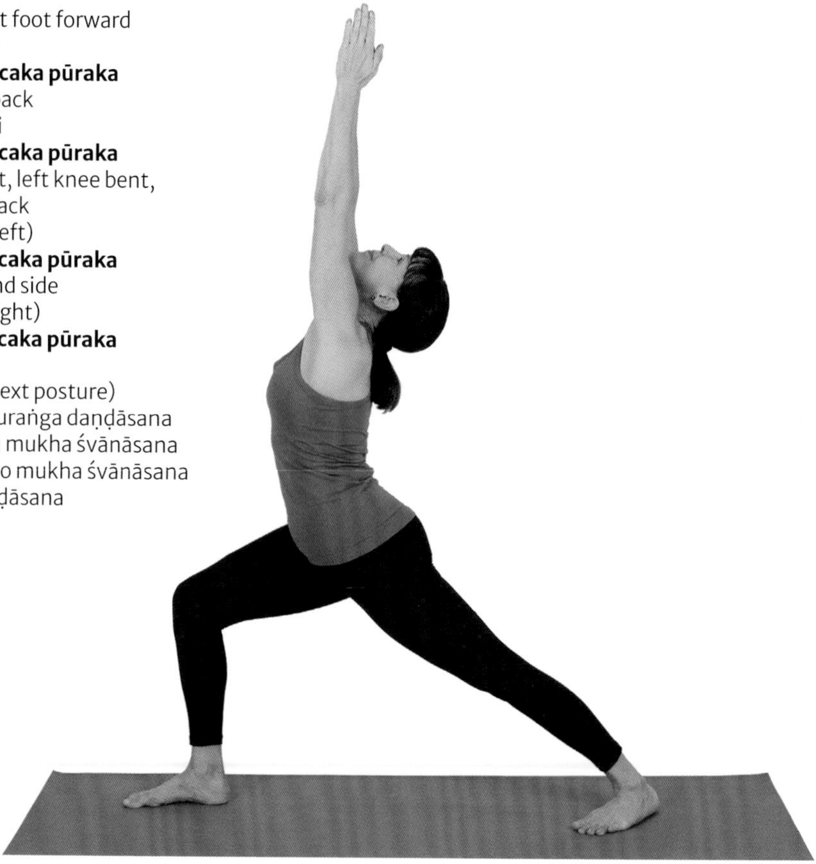

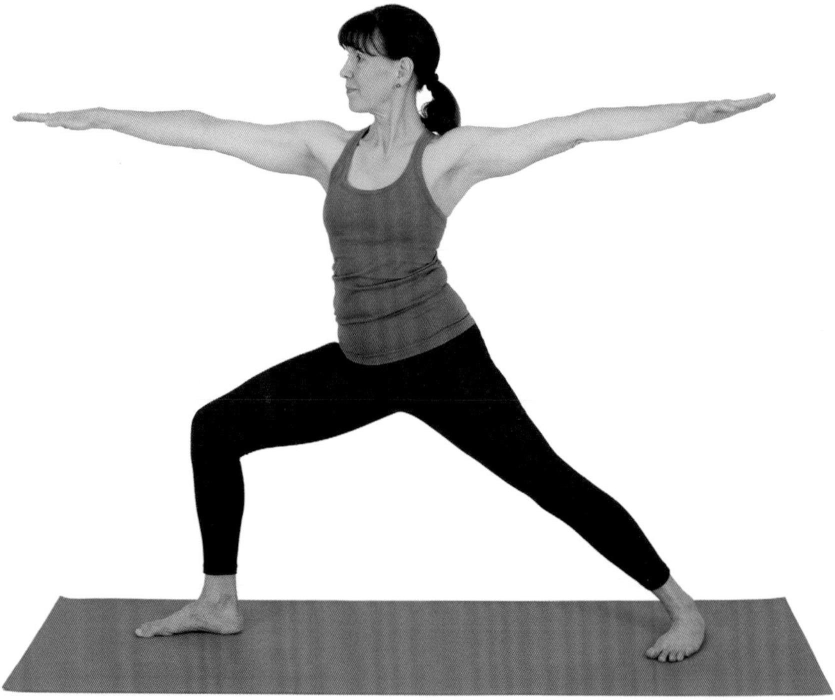

"The difference with Ashtanga is in the breath – you are ultimately learning to breathe. The purpose of the sounds of the breath is to quiet the mind and to generate heat in the body. This allows us to go through the sequences more safely. The primary series develops the bandhas and equal breath."

Manju Jois

## Daṇḍāsanam दण्डासनम्

**Nasāgra dṛṣṭi**
**Dīrgha recaka pūraka**

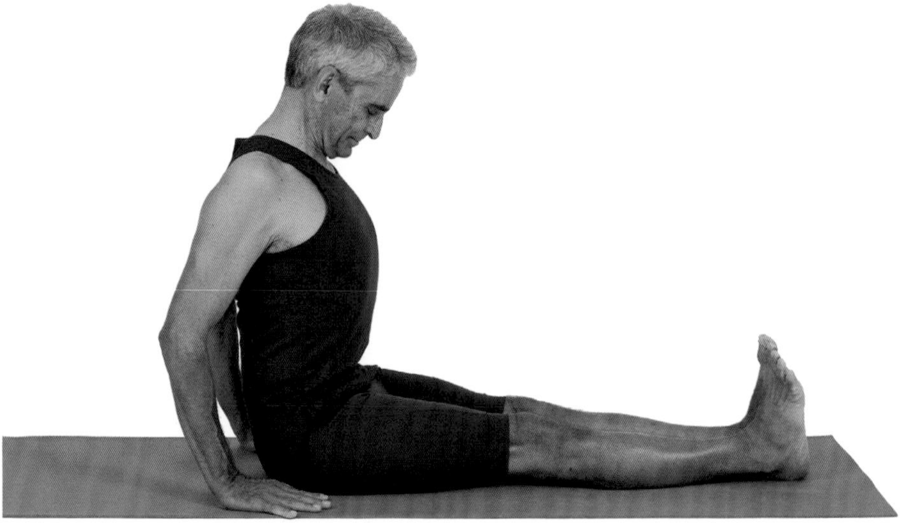

## Prathama Paścimatānāsanam प्रथम पश्चिमतानासनम्

**Ekam** - hold big toes with first two fingers and thumb, in
**Dwe** - ex, forward bend
**Nasāgra dṛṣṭi**
**Daśa dīrgha recaka pūraka**
**Trīṇi** - in, head up

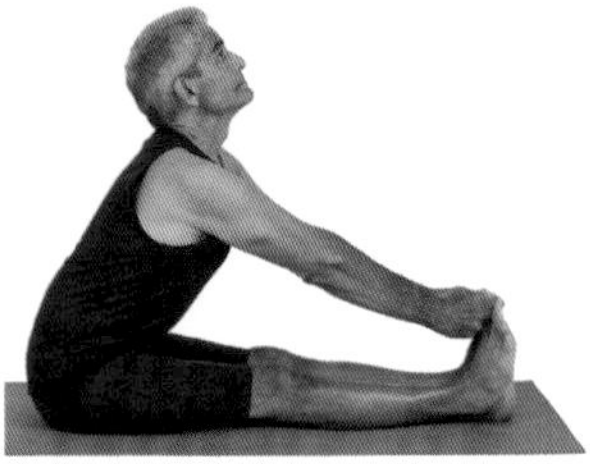

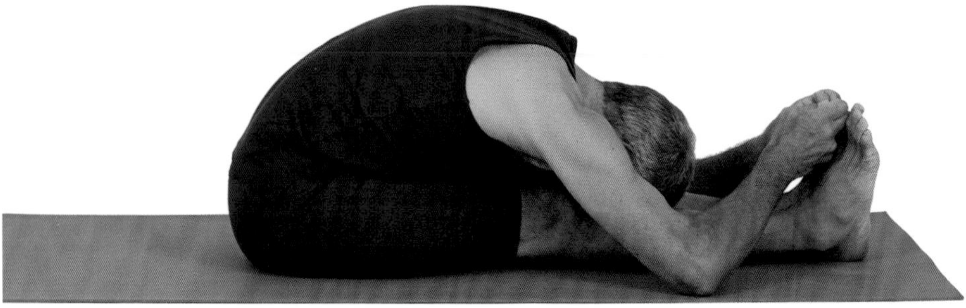

## Dwitīya Paścimatānāsanam द्वितीय पश्चिमतानासनम्

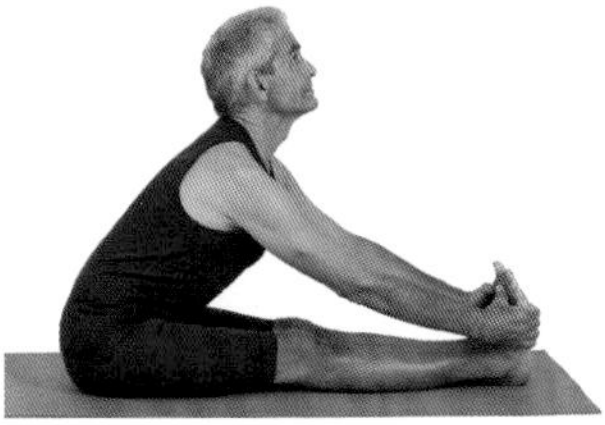

**Ekam** - hold sides of feet, in
**Dwe** - ex, forward bend
**Nasāgra dṛṣṭi**
**Daśa dīrgha recaka pūraka**
**Trīṇi** - in, head up

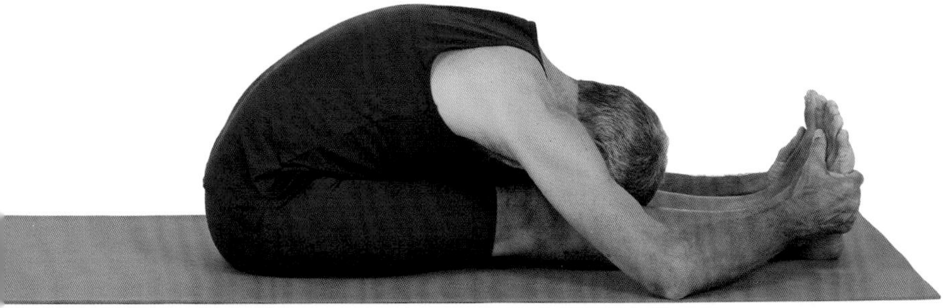

## Tṛtīya Paścimatānāsanam तृतीय पश्चिमतानासनम्

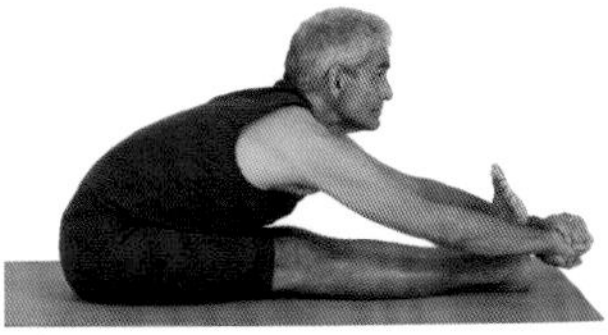

**Ekam** - left hand hold right wrist, in
**Dwe** - ex, forward bend
**Nasāgra dṛṣṭi**
**Daśa dīrgha recaka pūraka**
**Trīṇi** - in, head up
(transition to next posture)
**Catvāri** - ex, caturaṅga daṇḍāsana
**Pañca** - in, ūrdhva mukha śvānāsana
**Ṣat** - ex, adho mukha śvānāsana
**Sapta** - in, daṇḍāsana

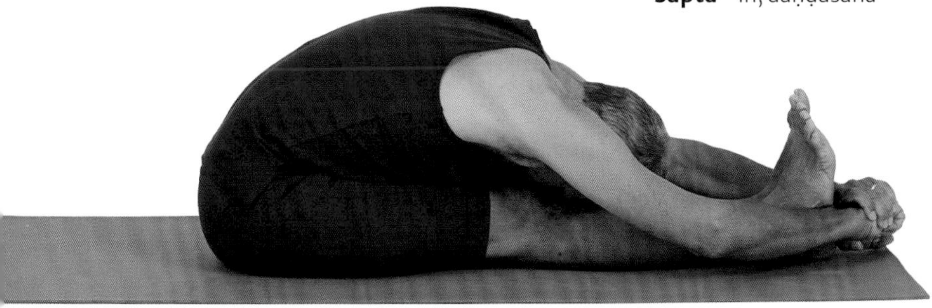

इति पश्चिमतानमासनाग्र्यं पवनं पश्चिमवाहिनं करोति ।
उदयं जठरानलस्य कुर्यादुदरे कार्श्यमरोगतां च पुंसाम् ॥ १:२९ ॥

Iti paścimatānamāsanāgyram pavanam paścimavāhinam karoti |
udayam jaṭharānalasya kuryādudare kārśyamarogatām ca pumsām || 1:29 ||

Thus, stay in this best back lengthened position, it carries energy (pavanam) to the back, raises the digestive fire, creates leanness in the belly, and lessens disease. HAṬHA YOGA PRADĪPIKĀ 1:29

**Ekam** - hands under shoulders

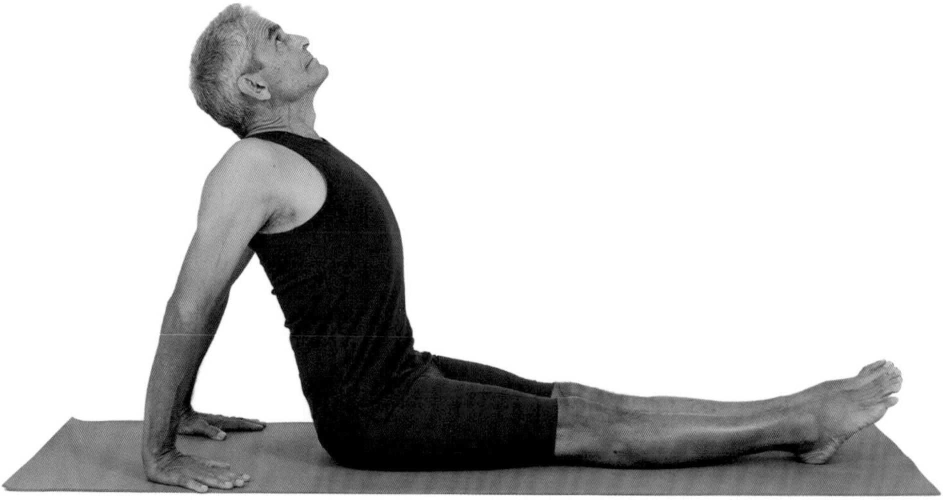

**Dwe** - in, come up
**Nasāgra dṛṣṭi**
**Daśa dīrgha recaka pūraka**
**Trīṇi** - ex, come down, in, utpluthiḥ
**Catvāri** - ex, caturaṅga daṇḍāsana
**Pañca** - in, ūrdhva mukha śvānāsana
**Ṣat** - ex, adho mukha śvānāsana
**Sapta** - in, daṇḍāsana

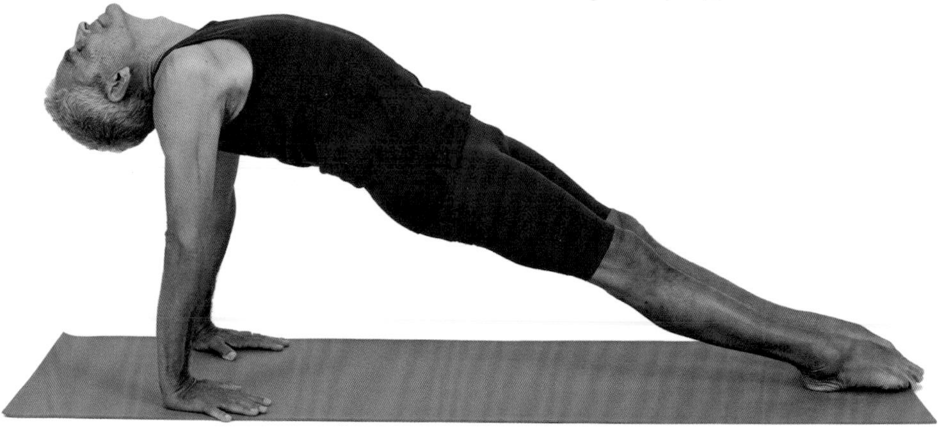

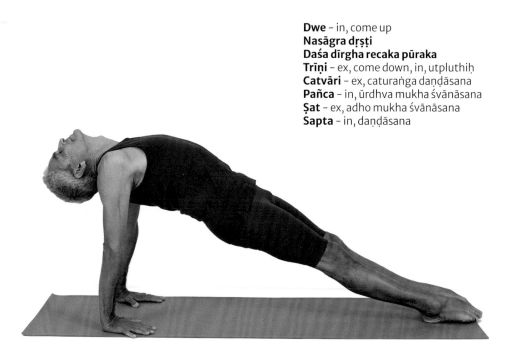

## Ardha Baddha Padma Paścimatānāsanam अर्ध बद्ध पद्म पश्चिमतानासनम्

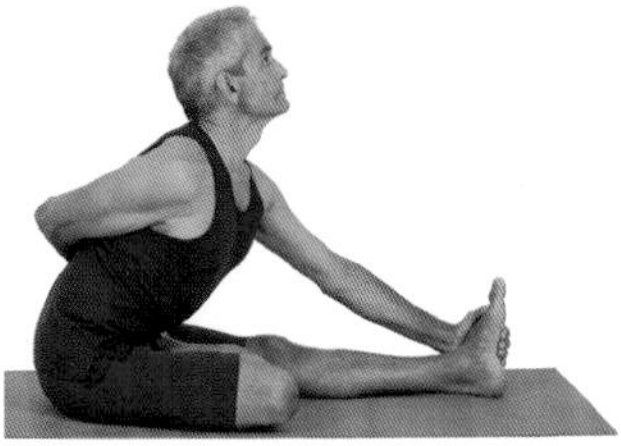

**Dakṣina bhāga**
**Ekam** – right foot half lotus, bind, left hand to front foot, in
**Dwe** – ex, forward bend
**Nasāgra dṛṣṭi**
**Daśa dīrgha recaka pūraka**
**Trīṇi** – in, head up, ex, utpluthiḥ, in
**Catvāri** – ex, caturaṅga daṇḍāsana
**Pañca** – in, ūrdhva mukha śvānāsana
**Ṣat** – ex, adho mukha śvānāsana
**Sapta** – in, daṇḍāsana
**Ardha Baddha Padma Paścimatānāsana**
**Wama bhāga**
(same as right side – Dakṣina bhāga)
(transition to next position)
**Catvāri** – ex, caturaṅga daṇḍāsana
**Pañca** – in, ūrdhva mukha śvānāsana
**Ṣat** – ex, adho mukha śvānāsana
**Sapta** – in, daṇḍāsana

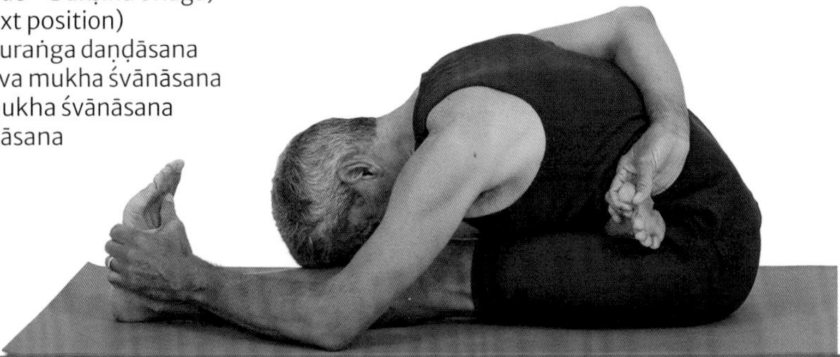

## Tiryañc Mukhaika Pāda Paścimatānāsasam तिर्यञ्च् मुखैक पाद पश्चिमतानासनम्

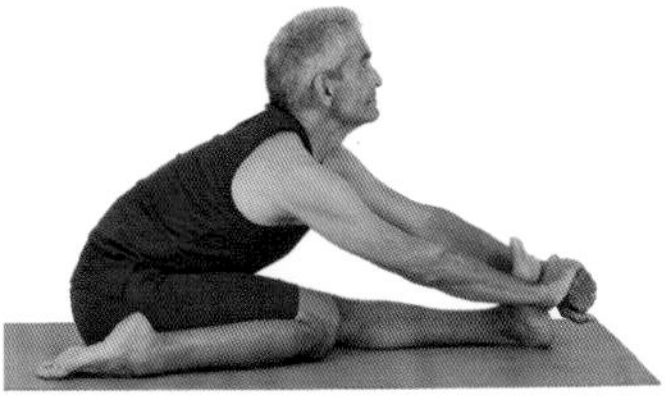

**Dakṣina bhāga**
**Ekam** – fold right leg, heel to outside of hip, bind foot, in
**Dwe** – ex, forward bend
**Nasāgra dṛṣṭi**
**Daśa dīrgha recaka pūraka**
**Trīṇi** – in, head up, ex, utpluthiḥ
**Catvāri** – ex, caturaṅga daṇḍāsana
**Pañca** – in, ūrdhva mukha śvānāsana
**Ṣat** – ex, adho mukha śvānāsana
**Sapta** – in, daṇḍāsana
**Tiryaṅg Mukhaika Pāda Paścimatānāsana**
**Wama bhāga**
(same as right side – Dakṣina bhāga)
(transition to next position)
**Catvāri** – ex, caturaṅga daṇḍāsana
**Pañca** – in, ūrdhva mukha śvānāsana
**Ṣat** – ex, adho mukha śvānāsana
**Sapta** – in, daṇḍāsana

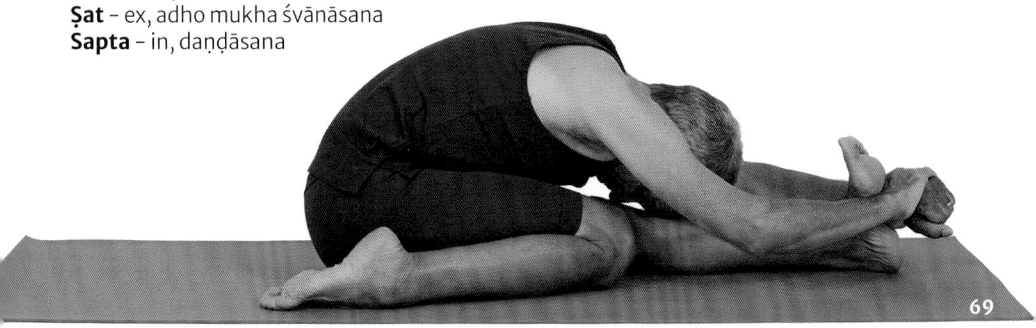

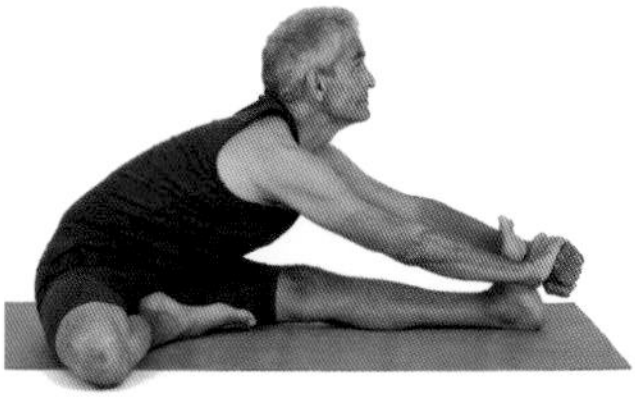

**Dakṣina bhāga**
**Ekam** - right heel to the groin, bind foot, in
**Dwe** - ex, forward bend
**Nasāgra dṛṣṭi**
**Daśa dīrgha recaka pūraka**
**Trīṇi** - in, head up, ex, utpluthiḥ, in
**Catvāri** - ex, caturaṅga daṇḍāsana
**Pañca** - in, ūrdhva mukha
**Ṣat** - ex, adho mukha śvānāsana
**Sapta** - in, daṇḍāsana
**Prathama Jānu Śīrṣāsana**
**Wama bhāga**
(same as right side - Dakṣina bhāga)
(transition to next posture)
**Catvāri** - ex, caturaṅga daṇḍāsana
**Pañca** - in, ūrdhva mukha śvānāsana
**Ṣat** - ex, adho mukha śvānāsana
**Sapta** - in, daṇḍāsana

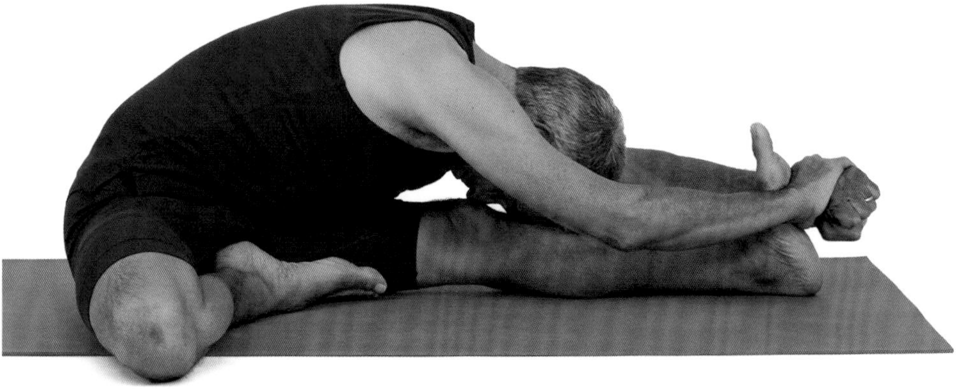

क्षयकुष्ठगुदावर्त्तगुल्माजीर्णपुरोगमाः ।
तस्य दोषाः क्षयं यान्ति महामुद्रां तु योऽभ्यसेत् ॥ ३:१७ ॥

Kṣayakuṣṭhagudāvarttagulmājīrṇapurogamāḥ |
tasya doṣāḥ kṣayam yāntimahāmudrām tu yo'bhyaset || 3:17 ||

From the practice of Mahāmudra (janū-śirṣāsana) there is relief from spleen or abdominal enlargement, digestive problems and diseases like Tuberculosis, Leprosy, & Piles.

HAṬHA YOGA PRAḌĪPIKĀ 3:17

## Dwitīya Jānu Śīrṣāsanam द्वितीय जानु शीर्षासनम्

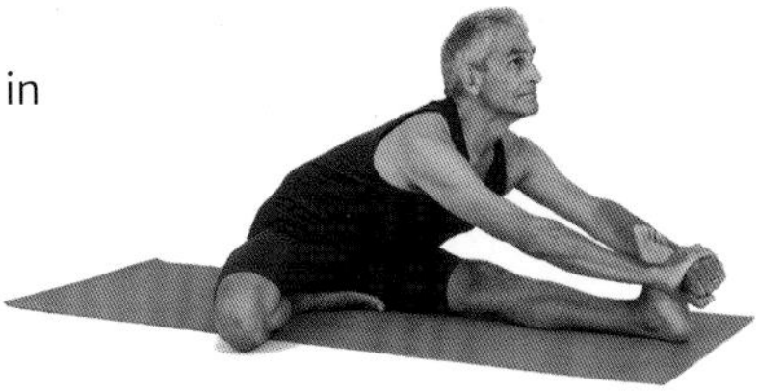

**Dakṣina bhāga**
**Ekam** – right heel under anus knee to side, bind foot, in
**Dwe** – ex, forward bend
**Nasāgra dṛṣṭi**
**Daśa dīrgha recaka pūraka**
**Trīṇi** – in, head up, ex, utpluthiḥ, in
**Catvāri** – ex, caturaṅga daṇḍāsana
**Pañca** – in, ūrdhva mukha śvānāsana
**Ṣat** – ex, adho mukha śvānāsana
**Sapta** – in, daṇḍāsana
**Dwitīya Jānu Śīrṣāsana**
**Wama bhāga**
(same as right side – Dakṣina bhāga)
(transition to next posture)
**Catvāri** – ex, caturaṅga daṇḍāsana

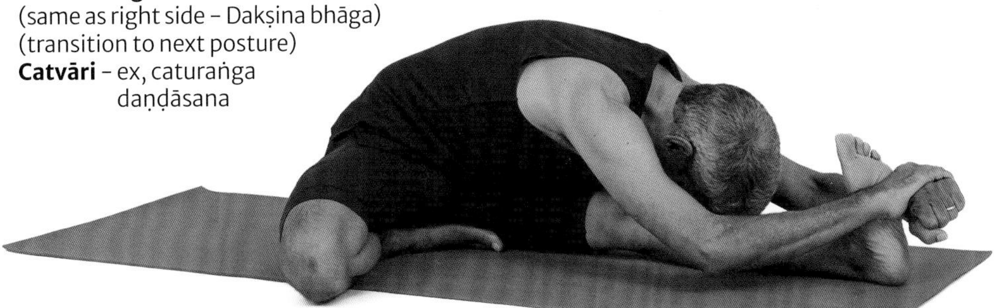

**Pañca** – in, ūrdhva mukha śvānāsana
**Ṣat** – ex, adho mukha śvānāsana
**Sapta** – in, daṇḍāsana

## Tṛtīya Jānu Śīrṣāsanam तृतीय जानु शीर्षासनम्

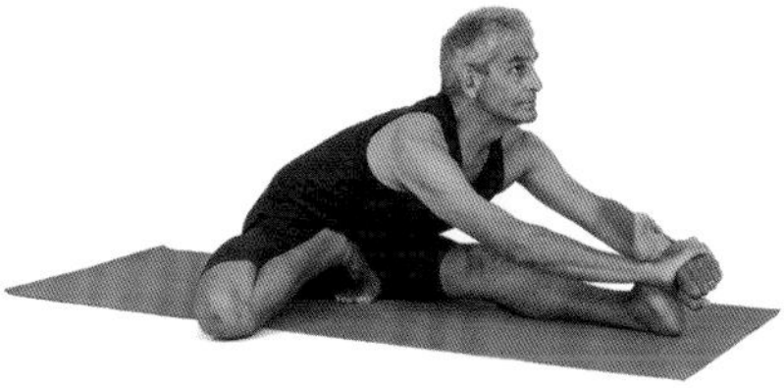

**Dakṣina bhāga**
**Ekam** – right foot flexed, ball of foot to floor, bind left foot, in
**Dwe** – ex, forward bend
**Nasāgra dṛṣṭi**
**Daśa dīrgha recaka pūraka**
**Trīṇi** – in, head up, ex, utpluthiḥ, in
**Catvāri** – ex, caturaṅga daṇḍāsana
**Pañca** – in, ūrdhva mukha śvānāsana
**Ṣat** – ex, adho mukha śvānāsana
**Sapta** – in, daṇḍāsana
**Tṛtīya Jānu Śīrṣāsana**
**Wama bhāga**
(same as right side – Dakṣina bhāga)
(transition to next position)
**Catvāri** – ex, caturaṅga daṇḍāsana
**Pañca** – in, ūrdhva mukha śvānāsana
**Ṣat** – ex, adho mukha śvānāsana
**Sapta** – in, daṇḍāsana

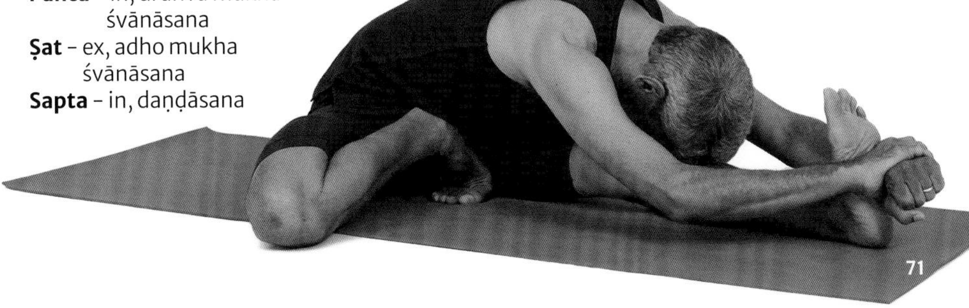

## Prathama Maricyāsanam   प्रथम मरिच्यासनम्

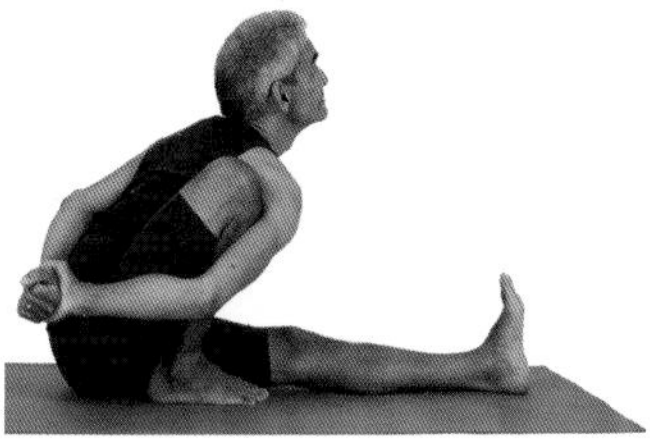

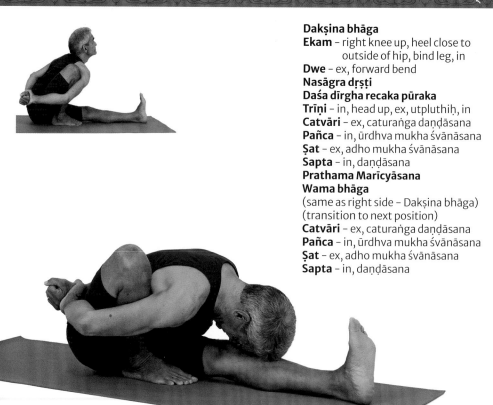

**Dakṣina bhāga**
**Ekam** - right knee up, heel close to outside of hip, bind leg, in
**Dwe** - ex, forward bend
**Nasāgra dṛṣṭi**
**Daśa dīrgha recaka pūraka**
**Trīṇi** - in, head up, ex, utpluthiḥ, in
**Catvāri** - ex, caturaṅga daṇḍāsana
**Pañca** - in, ūrdhva mukha śvānāsana
**Ṣat** - ex, adho mukha śvānāsana
**Sapta** - in, daṇḍāsana
**Prathama Marīcyāsana**
**Wama bhāga**
(same as right side - Dakṣina bhāga)
(transition to next position)
**Catvāri** - ex, caturaṅga daṇḍāsana
**Pañca** - in, ūrdhva mukha śvānāsana
**Ṣat** - ex, adho mukha śvānāsana
**Sapta** - in, daṇḍāsana

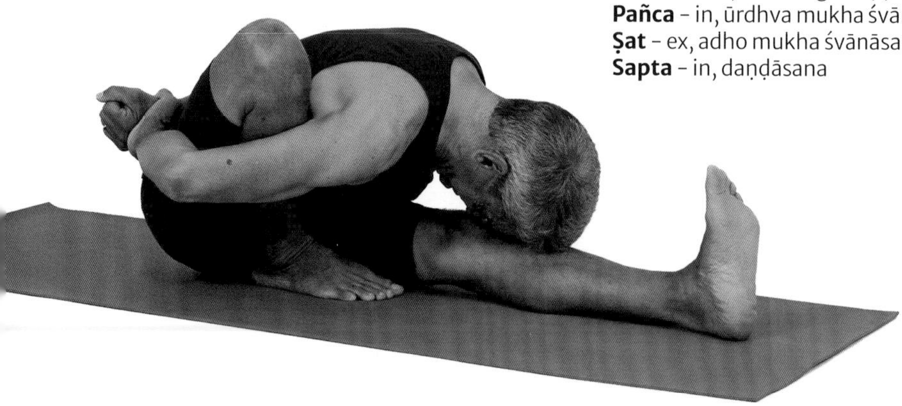

## Dwitīya Marīcyāsanam   द्वितीय मरीच्यासनम्

**Dakṣina bhāga**
**Ekam** - left leg half lotus, right knee up, heel close to outside of hip, bind leg, in
**Dwe** - ex, forward bend
**Nasāgra dṛṣṭi**
**Daśa dīrgha recaka pūraka**
**Trīṇi** - in, head up, ex, utpluthiḥ
**Catvāri** - ex, caturaṅga daṇḍāsana
**Pañca** - in, ūrdhva mukha śvānāsana
**Ṣat** - ex, adho mukha śvānāsana
**Sapta** - in, daṇḍāsana
**Dwitīya Marīcyāsana**
**Wama bhāga**
(same as right side - Dakṣina bhāga)
(transition to next position)
**Catvāri** - ex, caturaṅga daṇḍāsana
**Pañca** - in, ūrdhva mukha śvānāsana
**Ṣat** - ex, adho mukha śvānāsana
**Sapta** - in, daṇḍāsana

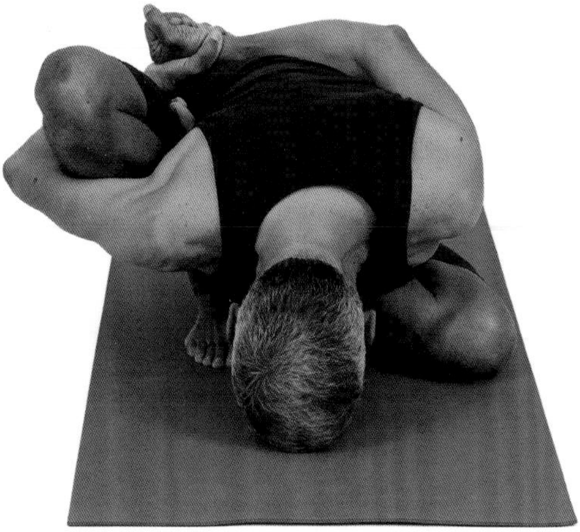

## Tṛtīya Marīcyāsanam

## तृतीय मरीच्यासनम्

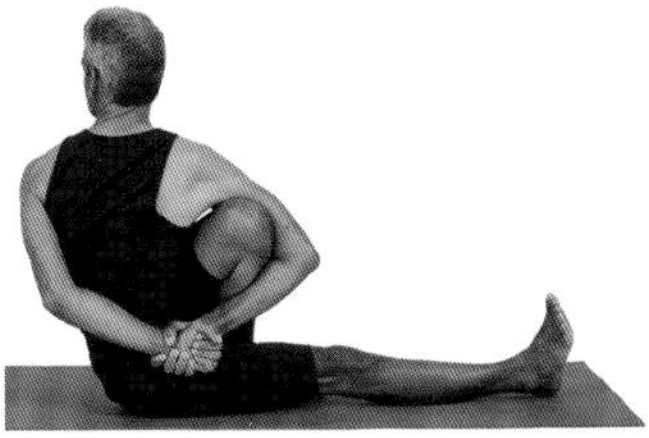

**Dakṣina bhāga**
**Ekam** - left straight, right bend, bring the shoulder to the outside side, in
**Dwe** - ex, bind and twist
**Pārśva dṛṣṭi**
**Daśa dīrgha recaka pūraka**
**Trīṇi** - release position, utpluthiḥ, in
**Catvāri** - ex, caturaṅga daṇḍāsana
**Pañca** - in, ūrdhva mukha śvānāsana
**Ṣat** - ex, adho mukha śvānāsana
**Sapta** - in, daṇḍāsana
**Tṛtīya Marīcyāsana**
**Wama bhāga**
(same as right side - Dakṣina bhāga)
(transition to next position)
**Catvāri** - ex, caturaṅga daṇḍāsana
**Pañca** - in, ūrdhva mukha śvānāsana
**Ṣat** - ex, adho mukha śvānāsana
**Sapta** - in, daṇḍāsana

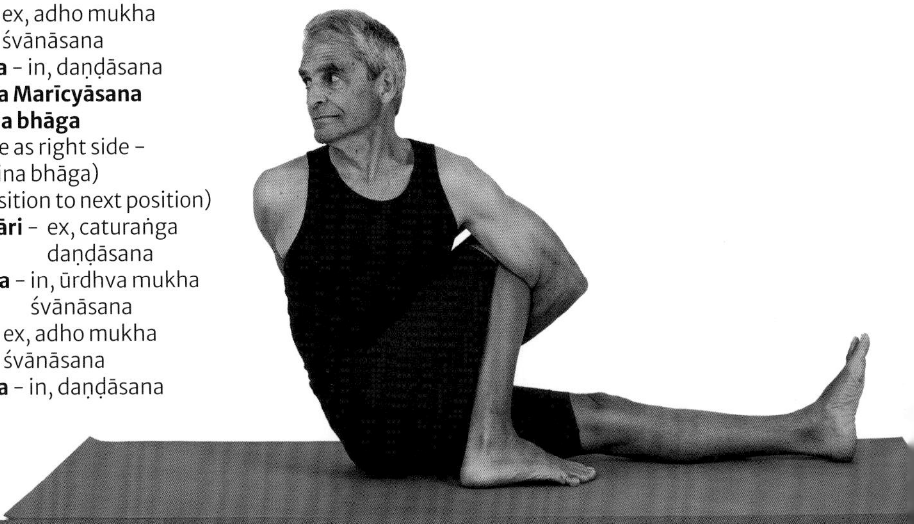

## Caturtha Marīcyāsanam

## चतुर्थ मरीच्यासनम्

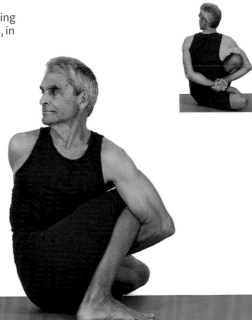

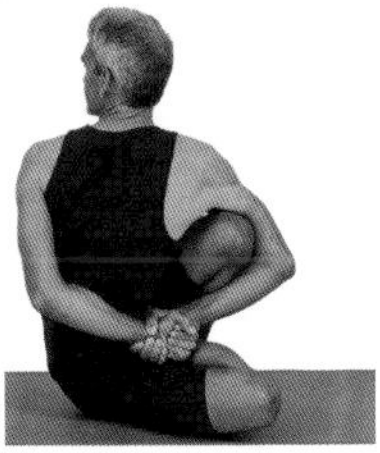

**Dakṣina bhāga**
**Ekam** - left leg half lotus, right bend, bring the shoulder to the outside side, in
**Dwe** - ex, bind and twist
**Pārśva dṛṣṭi**
**Daśa dīrgha recaka pūraka**
**Trīṇi** - release position, utpluthiḥ
**Catvāri** - ex, caturaṅga daṇḍāsana
**Pañca** - in, ūrdhva mukha śvānāsana
**Ṣat** - ex, adho mukha śvānāsana
**Sapta** - in, daṇḍāsana
**Caturtha Marīcyāsana**
**Wama bhāga**
(same as right side - Dakṣina bhāga)
(transition to next position)
**Catvāri** - ex, caturaṅga daṇḍāsana
**Pañca** - in, ūrdhva mukha śvānāsana
**Ṣat** - ex, adho mukha śvānāsana
**Sapta** - in, daṇḍāsana

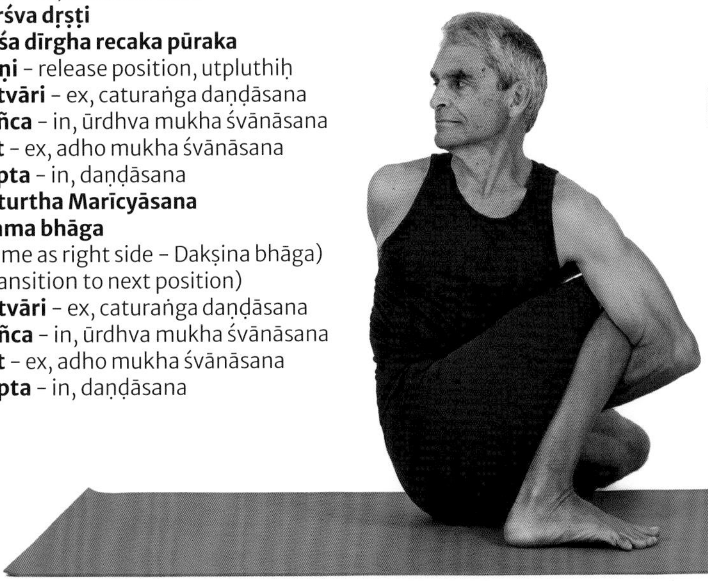

## Nāvāsanam नावासनम्

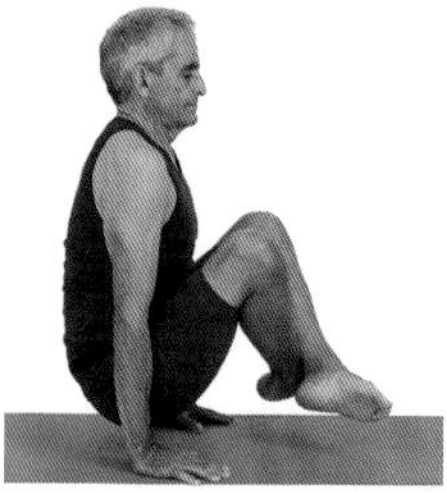
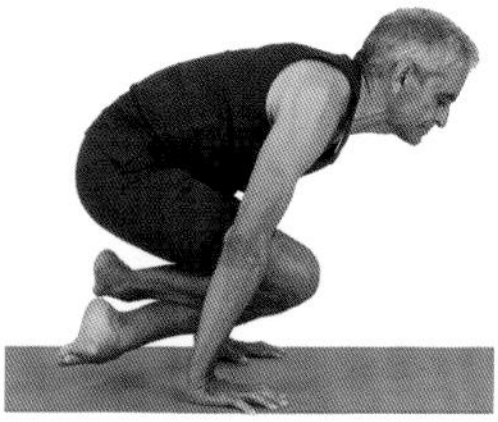

**Nāvāsanam** (lift the legs, hands beside the knees)
**Pādāṅguṣṭha dṛṣṭi**
**Daśa dīrgha recaka pūraka**
**Utpluthiḥ** - in
(repeat 3 -5 times)
(transition to next position)
**Catvāri** - ex, caturaṅga daṇḍāsana
**Pañca** - in, ūrdhva mukha śvānāsana
**Ṣat** - ex, adho mukha śvānāsana
**Sapta** - Bhujapīdāsana

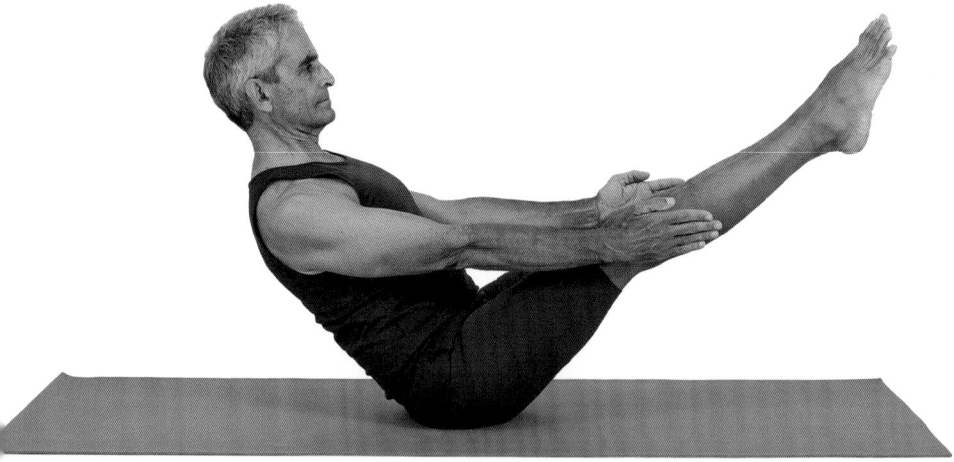

## Bhujapīḍāsanam भुजपीडासनम्

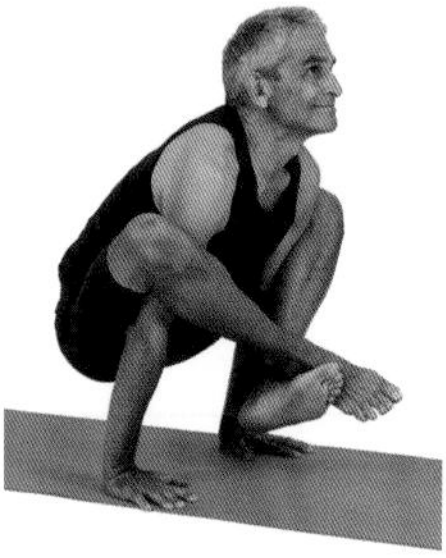

**Ekam** - jump legs around upper arms, right ankle crossed over left
**Dwe** - ex, head to the floor
**Nasāgra dṛṣṭi**
**Daśa dīrgha recaka pūraka**
**Trīṇi** - in, head up
(transition to next position)
**Catvāri** - ex, caturaṅga daṇḍāsana
**Pañca** - in, ūrdhva mukha śvānāsana
**Ṣat** - ex, adho mukha śvānāsana
**Sapta** - Kūrmāsana

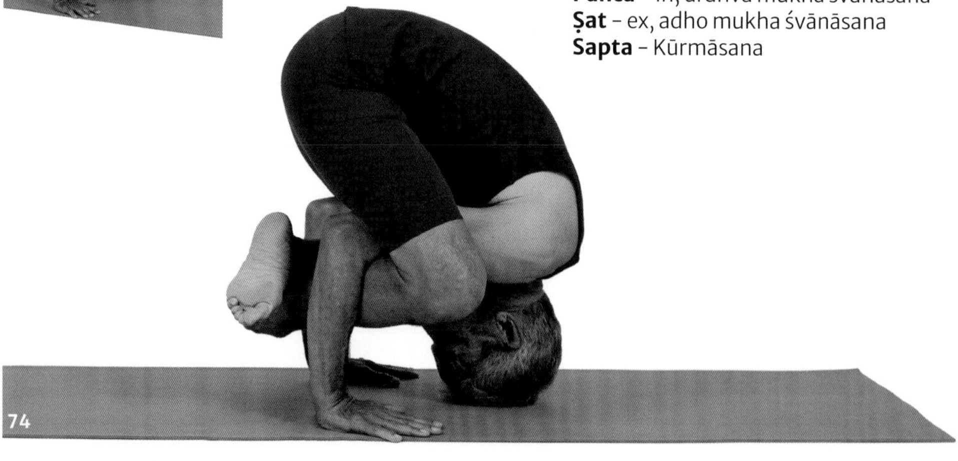

**Sapta** - jump knees over shoulders, stretch legs forward, arms to the sides
**Nasāgra dṛṣṭi**
**Daśa dīrgha recaka pūraka**

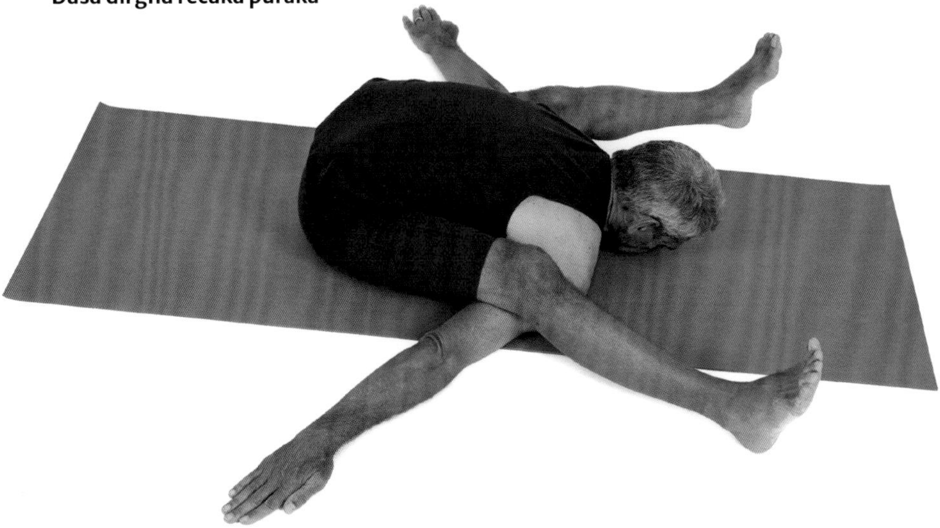

गुदं निरुध्य गुल्फाभ्यां व्युत्क्रमेण समाहितः ।
कूर्मासनं भवेदेतत् इति योगविदो विदुः ॥ १:२२ ॥

Gudam nirudhya guphābhyām vyutkrameṇa samāhitaḥ |
kūrmāsanam bhavedetat iti yogavido viduḥ || 1:22 ||

Constrain the anus by the ankles which move apart then come together. This is turtle position, indeed wise yogic knowledge. HAṬHA YOGA PRADĪPIKĀ 1:22

## Supta Kūrmāsanam सुप्त कूर्मासनम्

(Bind hands behind back, right foot over left)
**Nasāgra dṛṣṭi**
**Daśa dīrgha recaka pūraka**
**Trīṇi** - utpluthiḥ, in
(transition to next position)
**Catvāri** - ex, caturaṅga daṇḍāsana
**Pañca** - in, ūrdhva mukha śvānāsana
**Ṣat** - ex, adho mukha śvānāsana
**Sapta** - in, daṇḍāsana

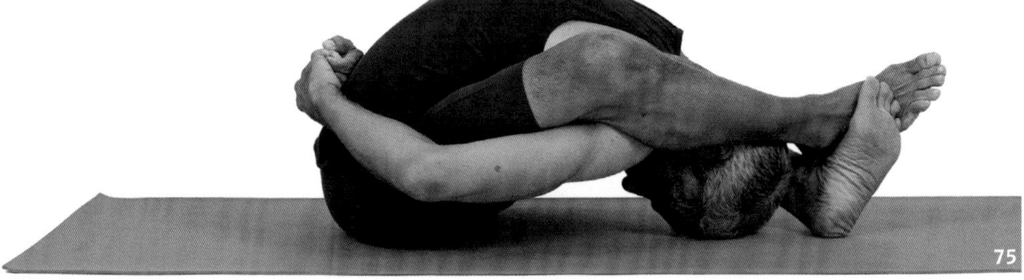

**Padmāsana**
(Insert arms between the thigh and the calf, hands to ears)
**Nasāgra dṛṣṭi**
**Daśa dīrgha recaka pūraka**
**Cakrāsana** – roll in circle, ex down, in up, roll up into Kukkuṭāsana

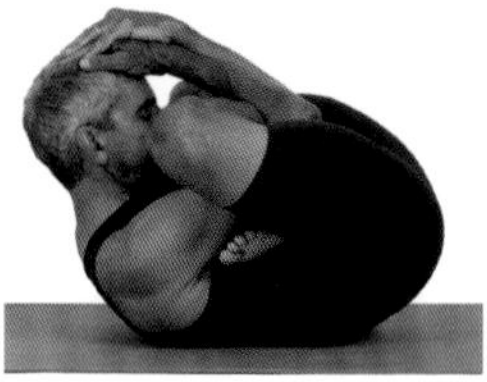

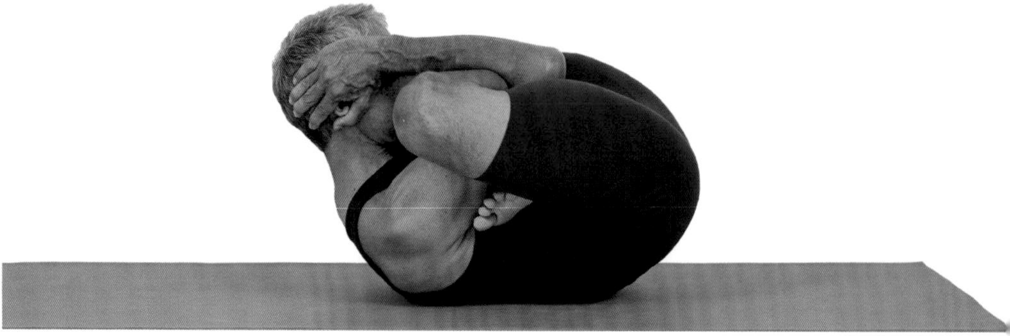

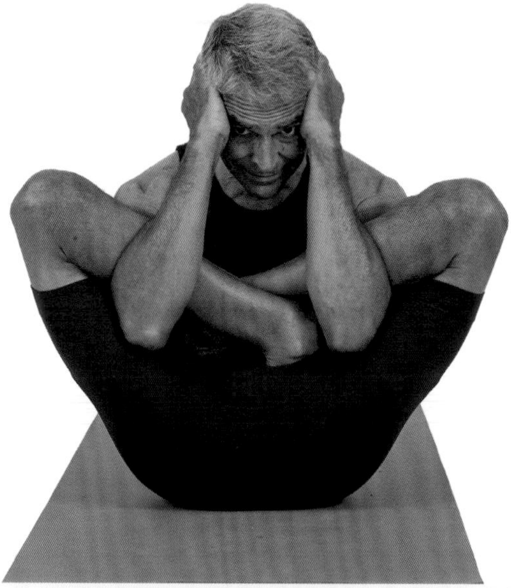

कुक्कुटासनबन्धस्थो दोर्भ्यां सम्बध्य कन्धराम् । भवेत्कूर्मवदुत्तान एतदुत्तानकूर्मकम् ॥ २:२४ ॥

Kukkuṭāsanabandhastho dorbhyām sambadhya kandharām |
bhavetkūrmavaduttāna etaduttānakūrmakam || 1:24 ||

Bind the Kukkuṭāsana by the forearms holding the head (and ears). Roll face up on the back. This resembles the shape of a Turtoise. HAṬHA YOGA PRADĪPIKĀ 1:24

**Ekam** - in, balance on the hands
**Daśa dīrgha recaka pūraka**
**Nasāgra dṛṣṭi**
**Dwe** - ex, come down
**Trīṇi** - utpluthiḥ, in
(transition to next position)
**Catvāri** - ex, caturaṅga daṇḍāsana
**Pañca** - in, ūrdhva mukha śvānāsana
**Ṣat** - ex, adho mukha śvānāsana
**Sapta** - in, daṇḍāsana

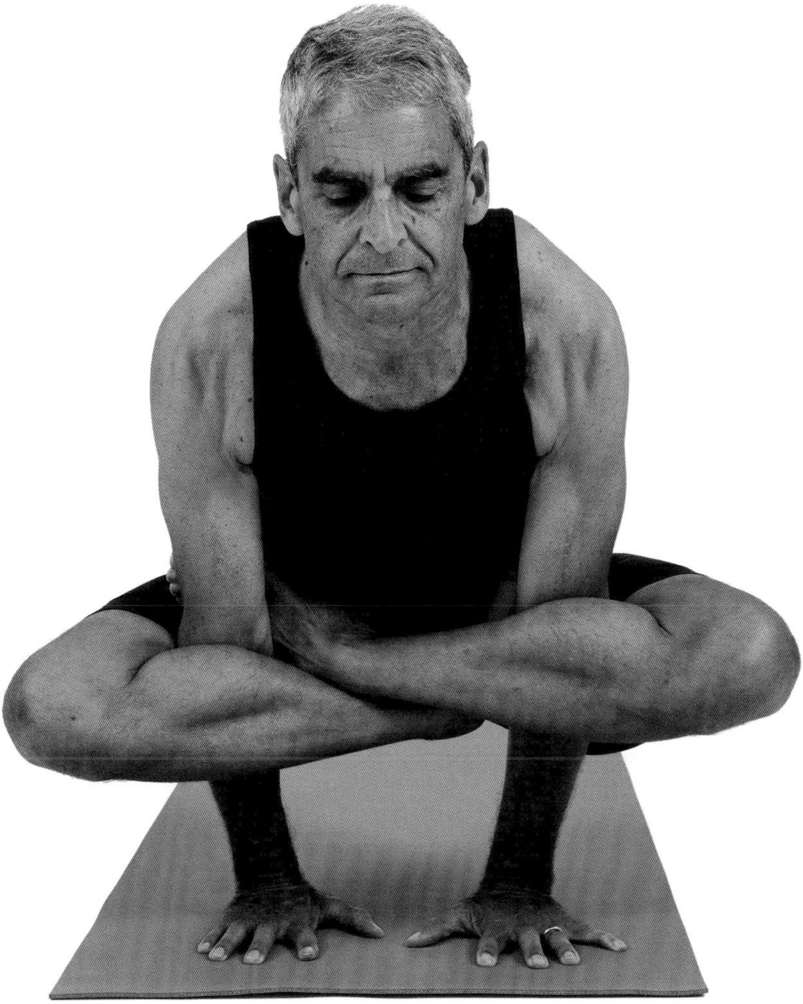

पद्मासनं तु संस्थाप्य जानूर्वोरन्तरे करौ ।
निवेश्य भूमौ संस्थाप्य व्योमस्थं कुक्कुटासनम् ॥ १:२३ ॥

Padmāsanam tu samsthāpya jānūrvorantare karau |
niveśya bhūmau samsthāpya vyomastham kukkuṭāsanam || 1:23 ||

Having come into Padmāsana (lotus position) insert the hands between the knees and thighs then entering the hands to the ground lift to the sky this is Kukkuṭāsaṇa. HAṬHA YOGA PRADĪPIKĀ 1:23

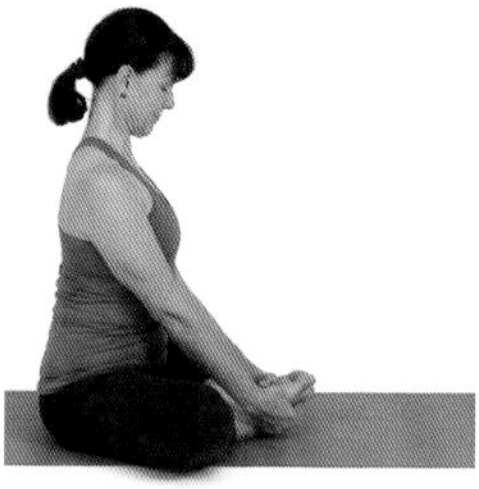

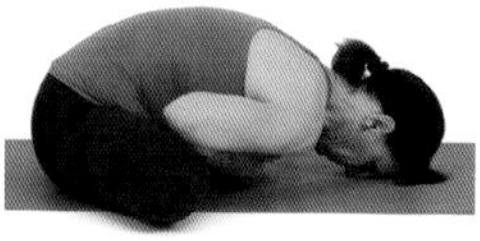

**Prathama Baddha Koṇāsana**
**Ekam** – bring heels close to the groin, hold feet
**Nasāgra dṛṣṭi**
**Daśa dīrgha recaka pūraka**
**Dwe** ex, head to floor
**Nasāgra dṛṣṭi**
**Daśa dīrgha recaka pūraka**
**Trīṇi** – in, come up
**Dwtīya Baddha Koṇāsana**
**Dwe** ex, crown of head to feet
**Nasāgra dṛṣṭi**
**Daśa dīrgha recaka pūraka**
**Trīṇi** – in, come up, ex, utpluthiḥ, in (transition to next position)
**Catvāri** – ex, caturaṅga daṇḍāsana
**Pañca** – in, ūrdhva mukha śvānāsana
**Ṣat** – ex, adho mukha śvānāsana
**Sapta** – in, daṇḍāsana

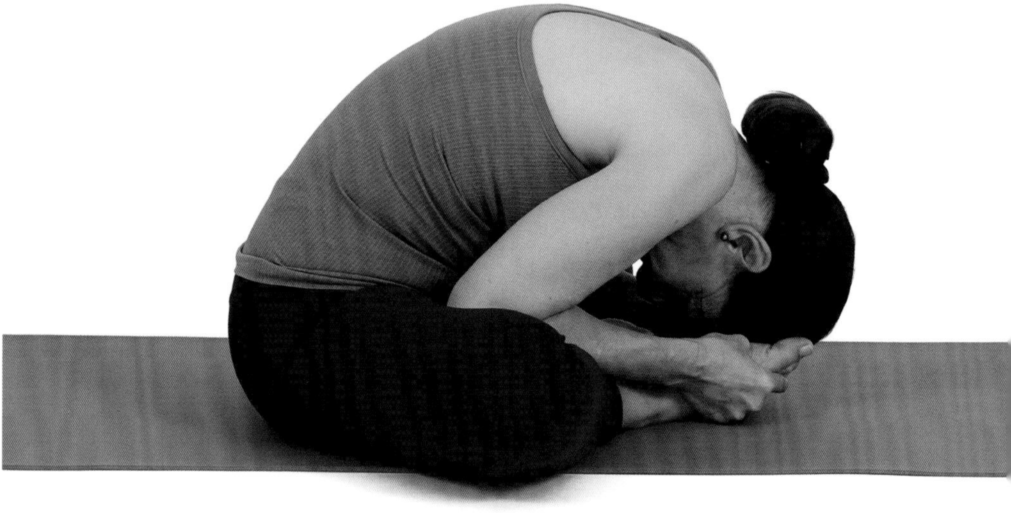

बद्धकोणासने तिष्ठं गुदमकुञ्चयेत् बुद्ध ।
गुदरोग्निवृत्तिः स्यात् सत्यं सत्यं ब्रविम्यहं ॥ वामन ऋषि

Baddhakoṇāsane tiṣtham gudamakuñcayet buddha |
gudarognivṛttiḥ syāt satyam satyam bravimyaham ||

Staying in Baddha koṇāsana contract the anus, it wards off disease in this area. This is the truth I declare. VĀMANA ṚṢI

## Upaviṣṭha Koṇāsanam उपविष्ठ कोणासनम्

**Ekam** - feet apart, hold big toes, head up, in
**Dwe** - ex, forward bend
**Nasāgra dṛṣṭi**
**Daśa dīrgha recaka pūraka**
**Trīṇi** - in, head up

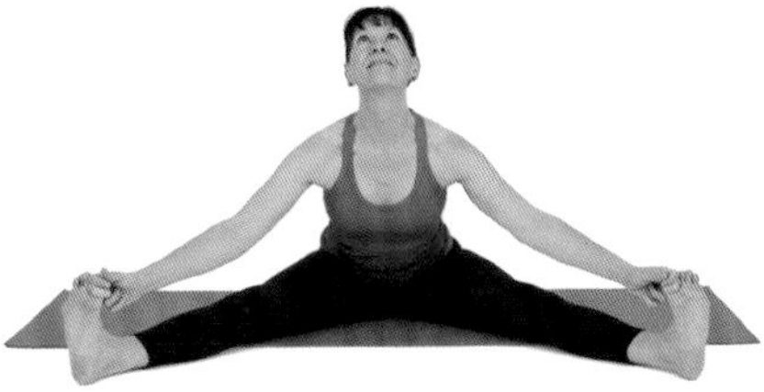

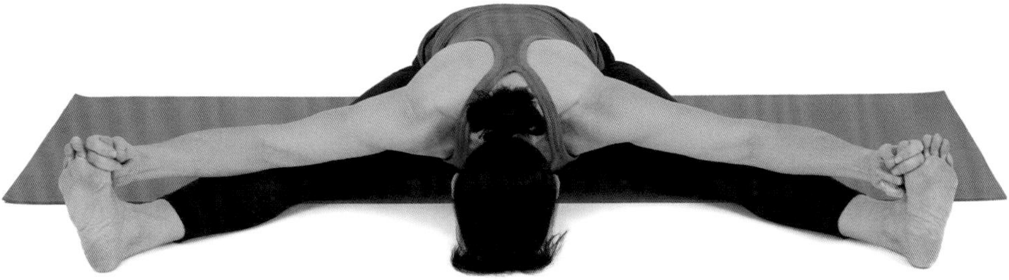

## Ūrdhva Mukha Upaviṣṭha Koṇāsanam ऊर्ध्व मुख उपविष्ठ कोणासनम्

(In, lift legs off floor, balance)
**Antarikṣa dṛṣṭi**
**Daśa dīrgha recaka pūraka**
(utpluthiḥ)
(transition to next position)
**Catvāri** - ex, caturaṅga daṇḍāsana
**Pañca** - in, ūrdhva mukha śvānāsana
**Ṣat** - ex, adho mukha śvānāsana
**Sapta** - in, daṇḍāsana, lie down

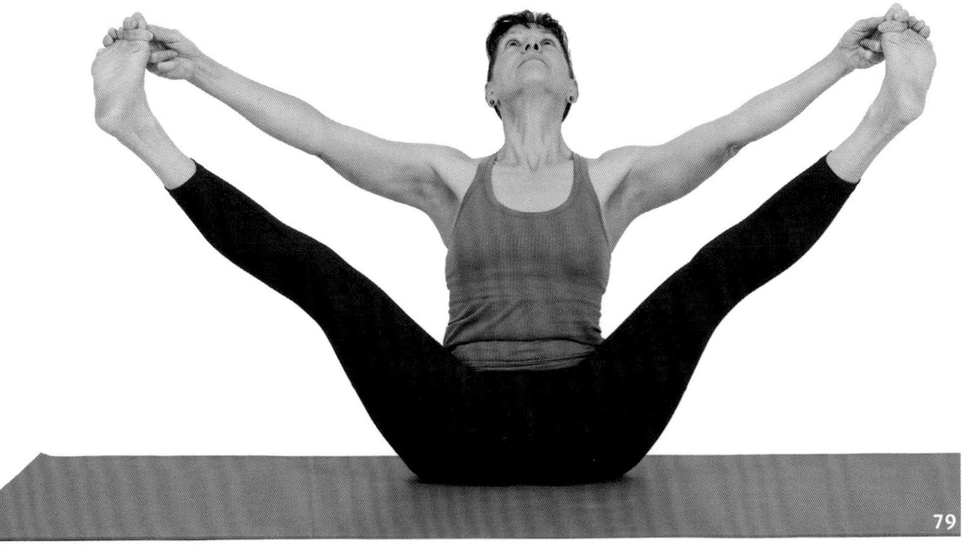

**Ekam** - in, both feet over the head, feet apart, hold big toes
**Nasāgra dṛṣṭi**
**Daśa dīrgha recaka pūraka**

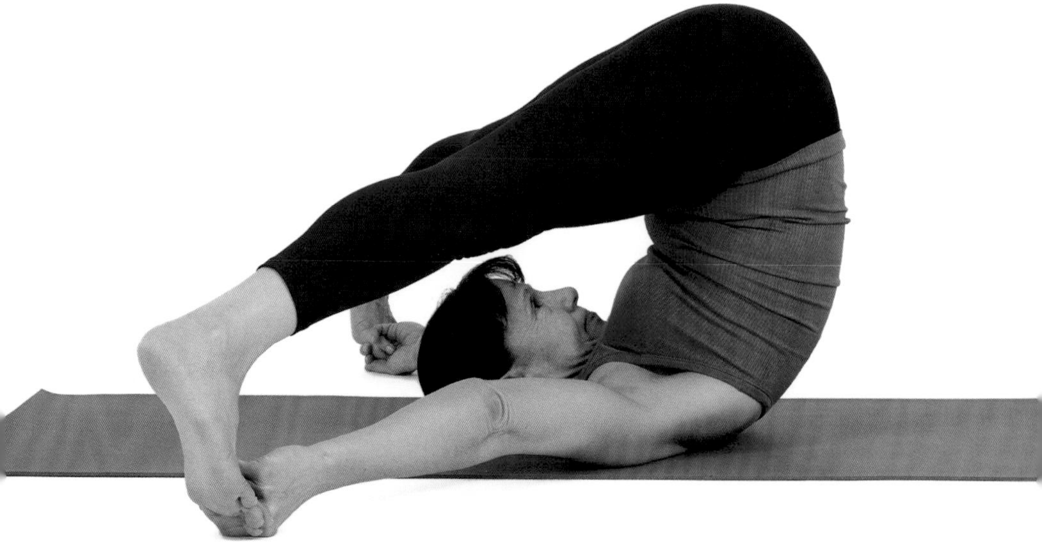

**Dwe** - in, roll legs to floor, head down, ex
**Trīṇi** - in, head up
(transition to next position)
(utpluthiḥ)
**Catvāri** - ex, caturaṅga daṇḍāsana
**Pañca** - in, ūrdhva mukha śvānāsana
**Ṣat** - ex, adho mukha śvānāsana
**Sapta** - in, daṇḍāsana, lie down

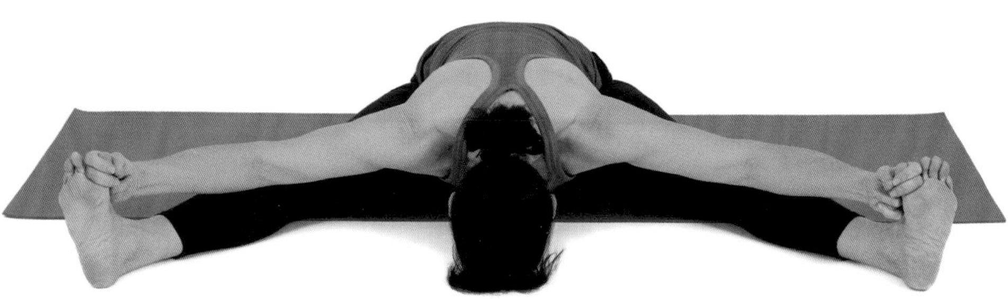

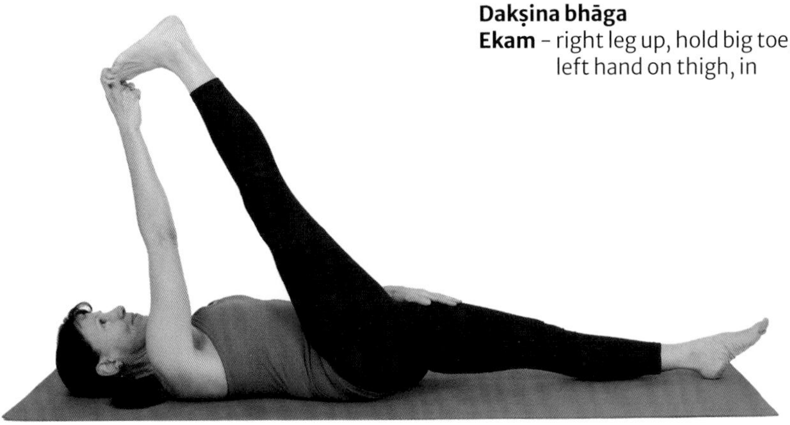

**Dakṣina bhāga**
**Ekam** - right leg up, hold big toe, left hand on thigh, in

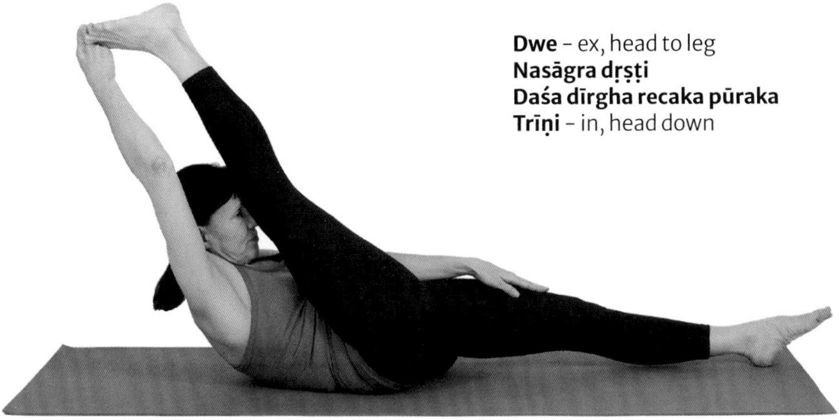

**Dwe** - ex, head to leg
**Nasāgra dṛṣṭi**
**Daśa dīrgha recaka pūraka**
**Trīṇi** - in, head down

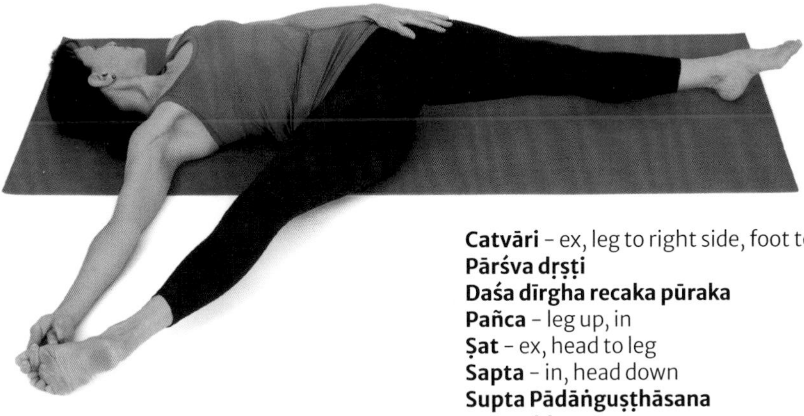

**Catvāri** - ex, leg to right side, foot to floor
**Pārśva dṛṣṭi**
**Daśa dīrgha recaka pūraka**
**Pañca** - leg up, in
**Ṣat** - ex, head to leg
**Sapta** - in, head down
**Supta Pādāṅguṣṭhāsana**
**Wama bhāga**
(same as right side - Dakṣina bhāga)
(transition to next position)
**Cakrāsana** - in, roll over the head (or sit up and jump back)
**Catvāri** - ex, caturaṅga daṇḍāsana
**Pañca** - in, ūrdhva mukha śvānāsana
**Ṣat** - ex, adho mukha śvānāsana

## Ubhaya Pādāṅguṣṭhāsanam उभय पादाङ्गुष्ठासनम्

**Ubhaya Pādāṅguṣṭhāsana**
**Ekam** - in, both feet to the floor behind head, hold toes
**Nasāgra dṛṣṭi**
**Daśa dīrgha recaka pūraka**

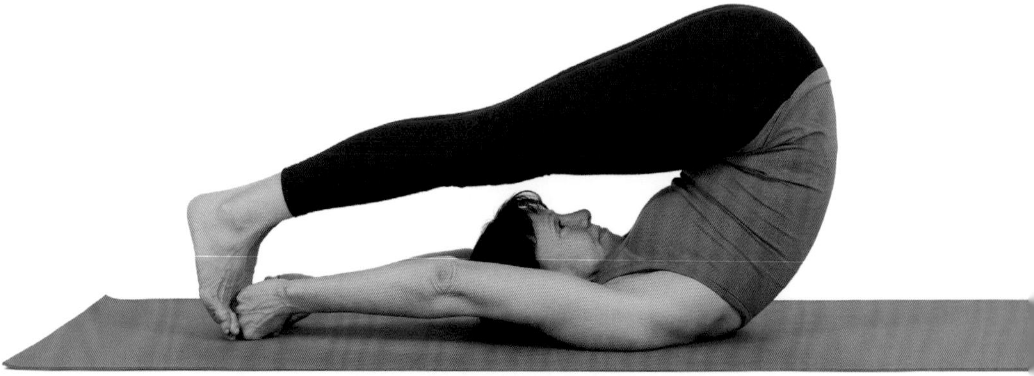

## Ūrdhva Pādāṅguṣṭhāsanam ऊर्ध्व पादाङ्गुष्ठासनम्

**Ūrdhva Pādāṅguṣṭhāsana**
**Dwe** - in, come up to balance
**Antarikṣa dṛṣṭi**
**Daśa dīrgha recaka pūraka**
**Trīṇi** - utplutiḥ, in
(transition to next position)
**Catvāri** - ex, caturaṅga dandāsana
**Pañca** - in, ūrdhva mukha śvānāsana
**Ṣat** - ex, adho mukha svānāsan
**Sapta** - in, daṇḍāsana

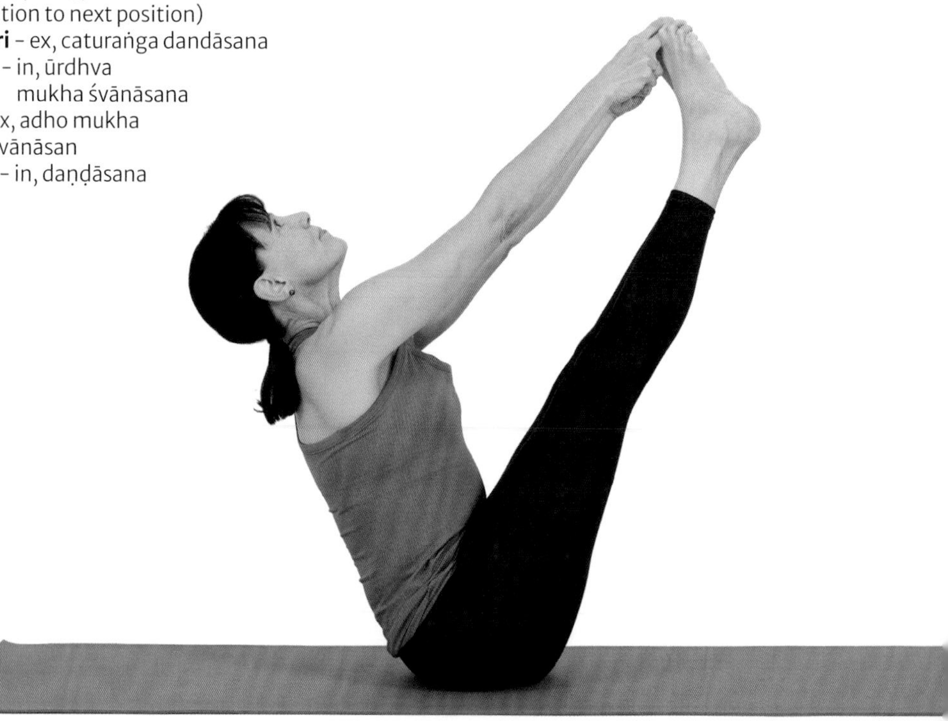

**Ekam** - in, both feet to the floor behind, ex, hold the feet
**Nasāgra dṛṣṭi**
**Daśa dīrgha recaka pūraka**

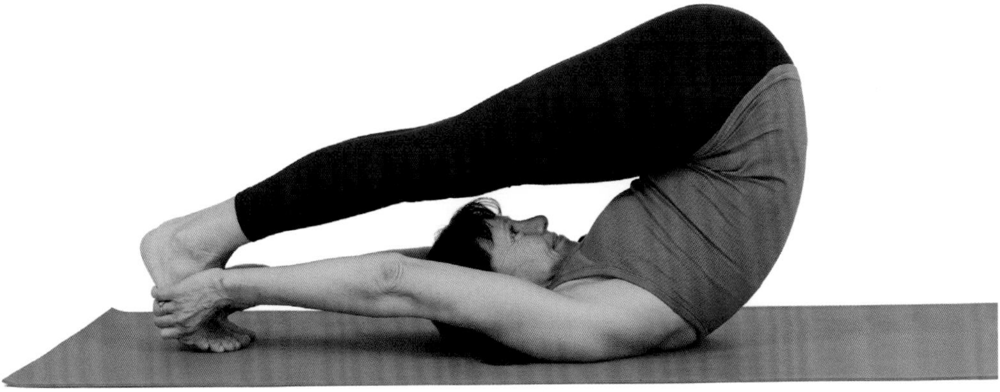

**Dwe** - in, come up balance on the hips, head the legs
**Nasāgra dṛṣṭi**
**Daśa dīrgha recaka pūraka**
**Trīṇi** - in, look up stretch arms (transition to next position) (utplutiḥ)
**Catvāri** - ex, caturaṅga daṇḍāsana
**Pañca** - in, ūrdhva mukha śvānāsana
**Ṣat** - ex, adho mukha śvānāsana
**Sapta** - in, daṇḍāsana, lie down

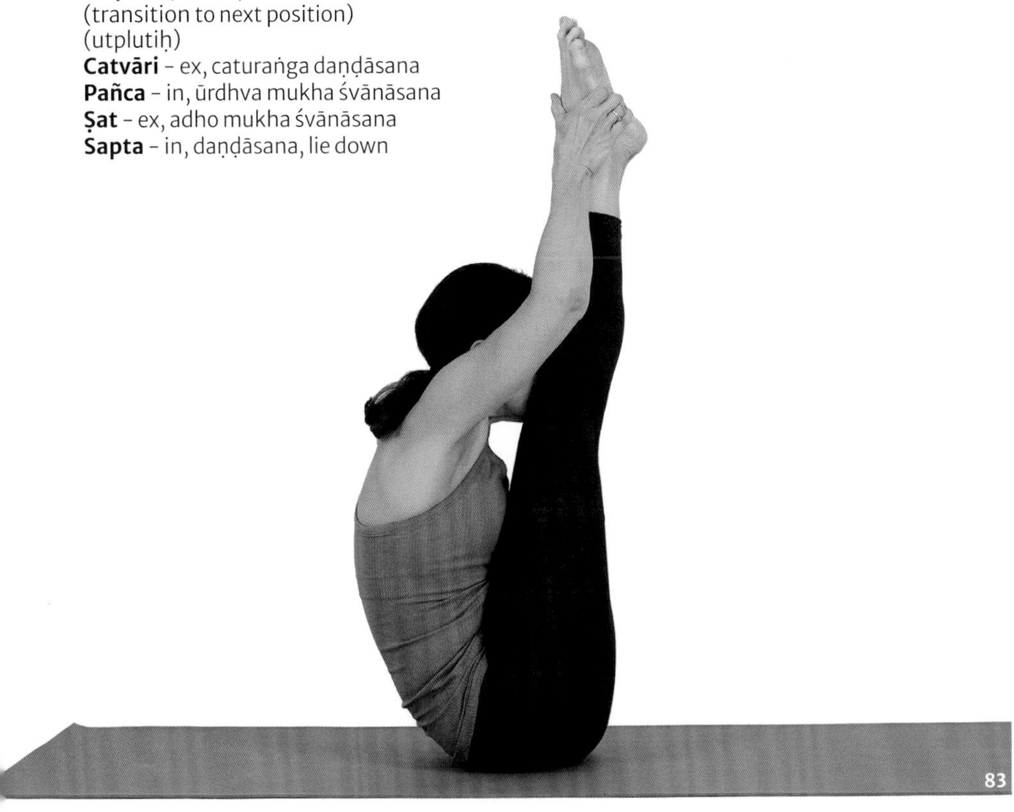

**Ekam** - bend knees slightly,
sides of the feet to floor,
place crown of head
on the floor,
fold arms across chest

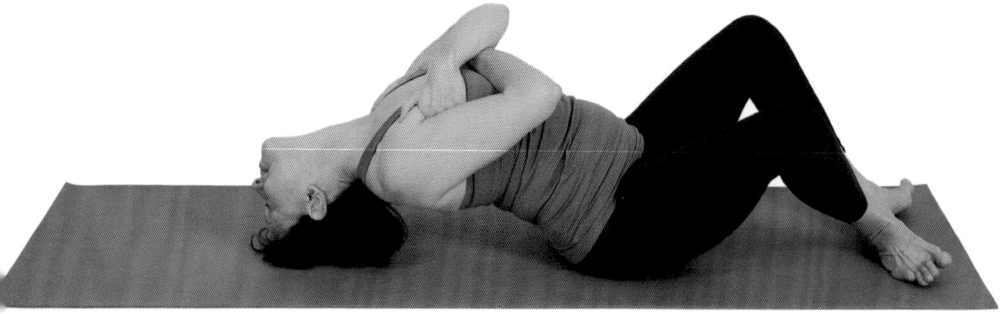

**Dwe** - in, stretch legs
**Nasāgra dṛṣṭi**
**Daśa dīrgha recaka pūraka**
**Trīṇi** - samasthitiḥ (lay down on back)
(transition to next position)
**Cakrāsana** - in, roll over the head
(or sit up and jump back)
**Catvāri** - ex, caturaṅga daṇḍāsana
**Pañca** - in, ūrdhva mukha śvānāsana
**Ṣat** - ex, adho mukha śvānāsana
**Sapta** - Pāśāsana

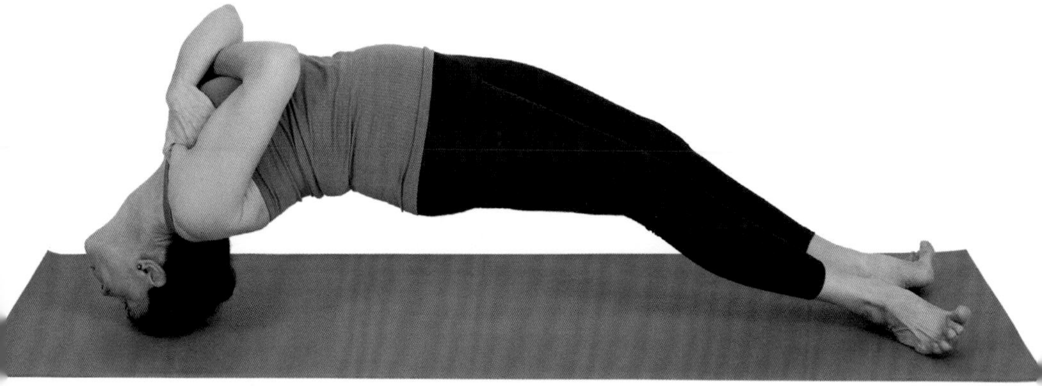

"Intermediate series works the meridians and the body at a deeper level, it stimulates the nervous system."

Manju Jois

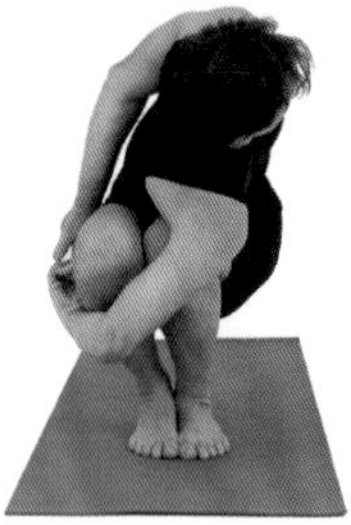

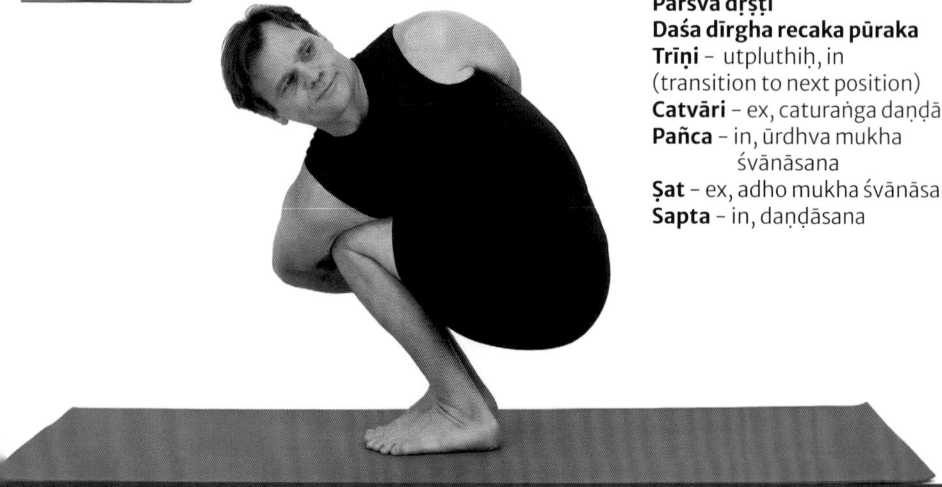

(Jump to squatting position hands)
**Dakṣina bhāga**
**Ekam** – ex, bind right leg, twist to the left
**Pārśva dṛṣṭi**
**Daśa dīrgha recaka pūraka**
**Wama bhāga**
(same as right side – Dakṣina bhāga)
**Dwe** – ex, bind left leg
**Pārśva dṛṣṭi**
**Daśa dīrgha recaka pūraka**
**Trīṇi** – utpluthiḥ, in
(transition to next position)
**Catvāri** – ex, caturaṅga daṇḍāsana
**Pañca** – in, ūrdhva mukha śvānāsana
**Ṣat** – ex, adho mukha śvānāsana
**Sapta** – in, daṇḍāsana

## Krauñcāsanam क्रौंचासनम्

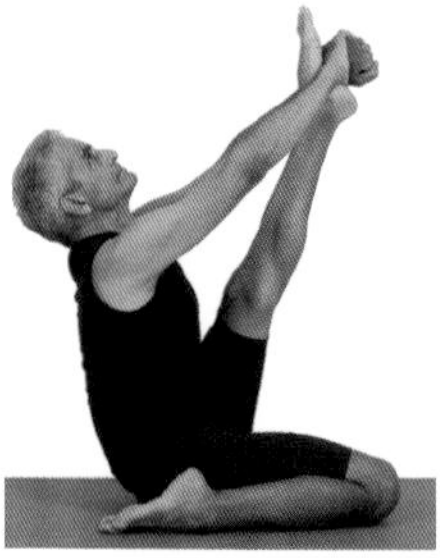

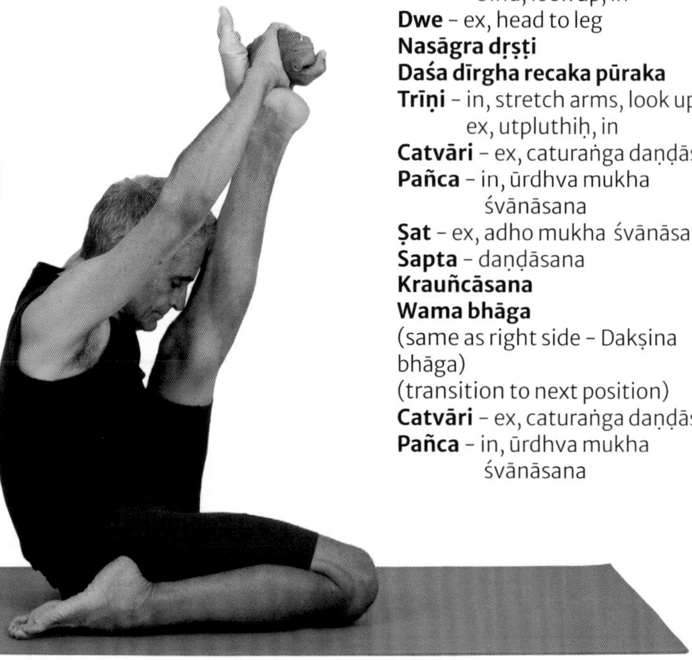

**Dakṣina bhāga**
**Ekam** – right leg bent, left leg up bind, look up, in
**Dwe** – ex, head to leg
**Nasāgra dṛṣṭi**
**Daśa dīrgha recaka pūraka**
**Trīṇi** – in, stretch arms, look up, ex, utpluthiḥ, in
**Catvāri** – ex, caturaṅga daṇḍāsana
**Pañca** – in, ūrdhva mukha śvānāsana
**Ṣat** – ex, adho mukha śvānāsana
**Sapta** – daṇḍāsana
**Krauñcāsana**
**Wama bhāga**
(same as right side – Dakṣina bhāga)
(transition to next position)
**Catvāri** – ex, caturaṅga daṇḍāsana
**Pañca** – in, ūrdhva mukha śvānāsana

## Prathama Śalabhāsanam

**Catvāri** - ex, caturaṅga daṇḍāsana

**Ekam** - place body to floor
**Dwe** - lift head and legs
**Nasāgra dṛṣṭi**
**Daśa dīrgha recaka pūraka**

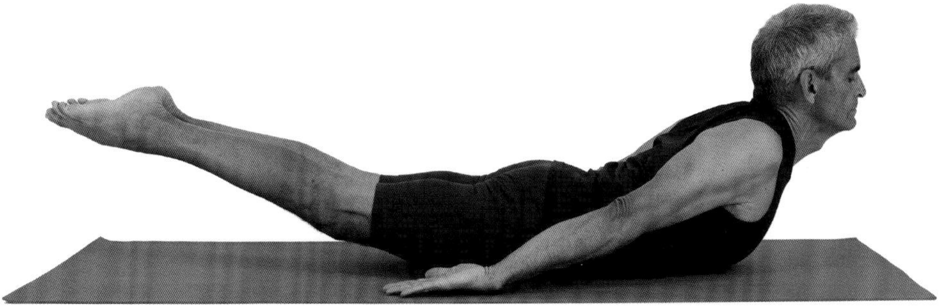

अध्यास शेते करयुग्मवक्ष आलम्भ्य भूमि करयोस्तलाभ्याम् ।
पादौ च शुन्ये च वितस्ति चोर्ध्वम् वदन्ति पीठं शलभं मुनीन्द्राः॥ २:३९ ॥

Adhyāsya śete karayugmavakṣa ālambya bhūmi karayostalābhyām |
pādau ca śūnye ca vitasti cordhvam vadanti pītam śalabham munīndrāḥ || 2:39 ||

Lay down in a sleeping position (on stomach) hands by the chest with both palms resting on the floor. The legs are extended into the void (above the body) lifted the height of Vitasti (the extended length between tip of thumb and little finger). This is called by the sages Śalabha the locust.

GHERAṆḌA SAMHITA 2:39

## Dwitīya Śalabhāsanam दितीय शलभासनम्

(Hands on floor beside waist)
**Nasāgra dṛṣṭi**
**Daśa dīrgha recaka pūraka**
(transition to next position)
**Pañca** - in, ūrdhva mukha śvānāsana
**Ṣat** - ex, adho mukha

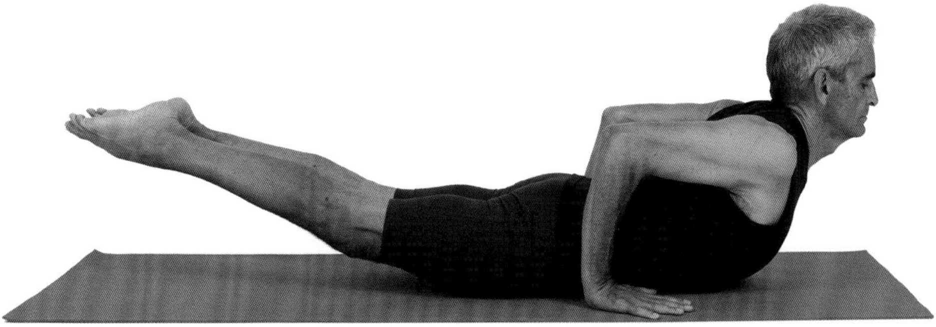

**Catvāri** - ex, caturāṅga daṇḍāsana

**Ekam** - śalabhāsana position hold feet
**Dwe** - in, head up press feet to floor
**Nasāgra dṛṣṭi**
**Daśa dīrgha recaka pūraka**
**Trīṇi** - ex, caturāṅga daṇḍāsana
(transition to next position)
**Catvāri** - in, ūrdhva mukha śvānāsana
**Pañca** - ex, adho mukha śvānāsana

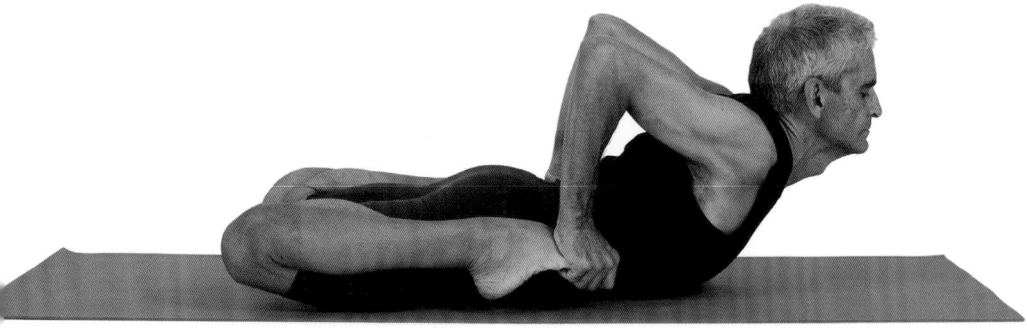

## Dhanurāsanam धनुरासनम्

**Catvāri** - ex, caturāṅga daṇḍāsana

**Ekam** - hold ankles
**Dwe** - in, come up
**Nasāgra dṛṣṭi**
**Daśa dīrgha recaka pūraka**
**Trīṇi** - ex, come down
(transition to next position)
**Catvāri** - caturāṅga daṇḍāsana
**Pañca** - ex, adho
mukha śvānāsana
**Ṣat** - adho mukha śvānāsana

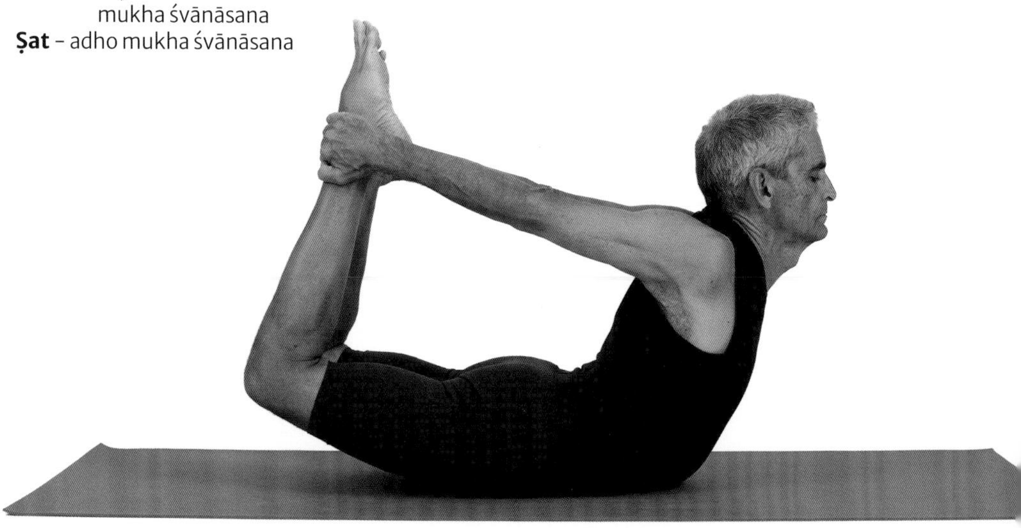

**Catvāri** – ex, caturāṅga daṇḍāsana

**Ekam** – hold ankles, in, come up
**Dwe** – ex, roll to the right
**Antarikṣa / ūrdhva dṛṣṭi**
**Daśa dīrgha recaka pūraka**
**Trīṇi** – in, come up, ex,
roll onto left side
**Antarikṣa/ūrdhva dṛṣṭi**
**Daśa dīrgha recaka pūraka**
**Catvāri** – in, come up
**Nasāgra dṛṣṭi**
**Daśa dīrgha recaka pūraka**
**Pañca** – ex, come down, caturaṅga daṇḍāsana
(transition to next position)
**Ṣat** – in, ūrdhva mukha śvānāsana
**Sapta** – ex, adho mukha śvānāsana

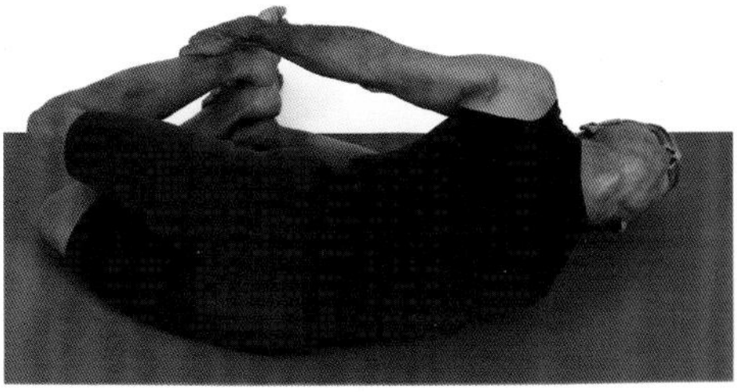

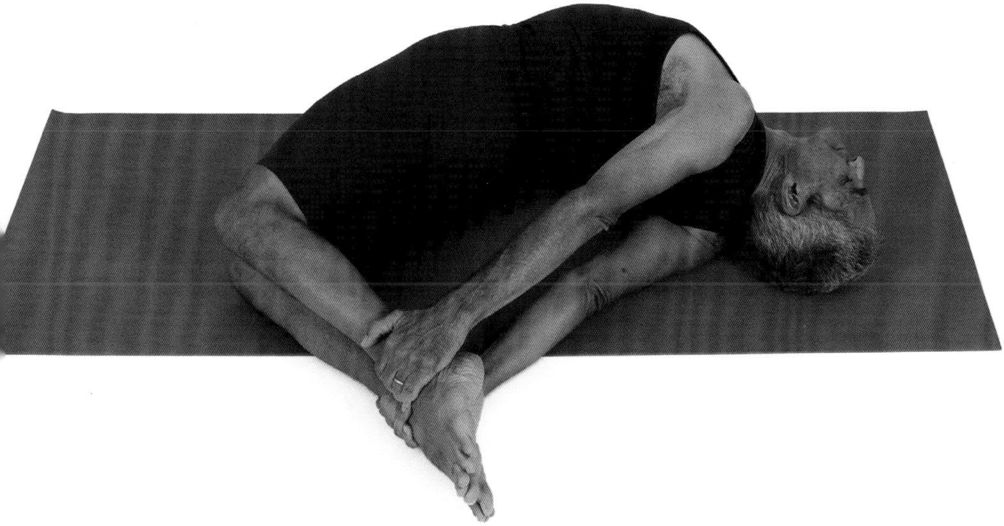

पादांगुष्टौ तु पाणिभ्यां गृहीत्वा श्रवणावधि ।
धनुराकर्षणं कुर्याद् धनुरासनमुच्यते ॥ १:२५ ॥

Pādāṅguṣṭau tu pāṇibhyām gṛhītvā śravaṇāvadhi |
dhanurākarṣaṇam kuryād dhanurāsanamucyate || 1:25 ||

With both hands grasp the ankles (or big toes) and bring them to the ears.
Having drawn tight the bow it is called Dhanurāsana. Haṭha Yoga Pradīpikā 1:25

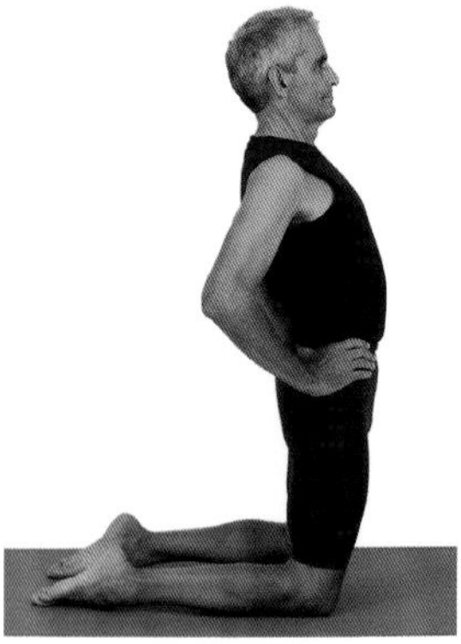

**Ekam** - knees hip width, hands on waist, in
**Dwe** - ex, hands to feet
**Nasāgra dṛṣṭi**
**Daśa dīrgha recaka pūraka**
**Trīṇi** - in, come up, ex, utpluthiḥ, in (transition to next position)
**Catvāri** - ex, caturaṅga daṇḍāsana
**Pañca** - in, ūrdhva mukha śvānāsana
**Ṣat** - ex, adho mukha śvānāsana
**Sapta** - Laghu vajrāsana

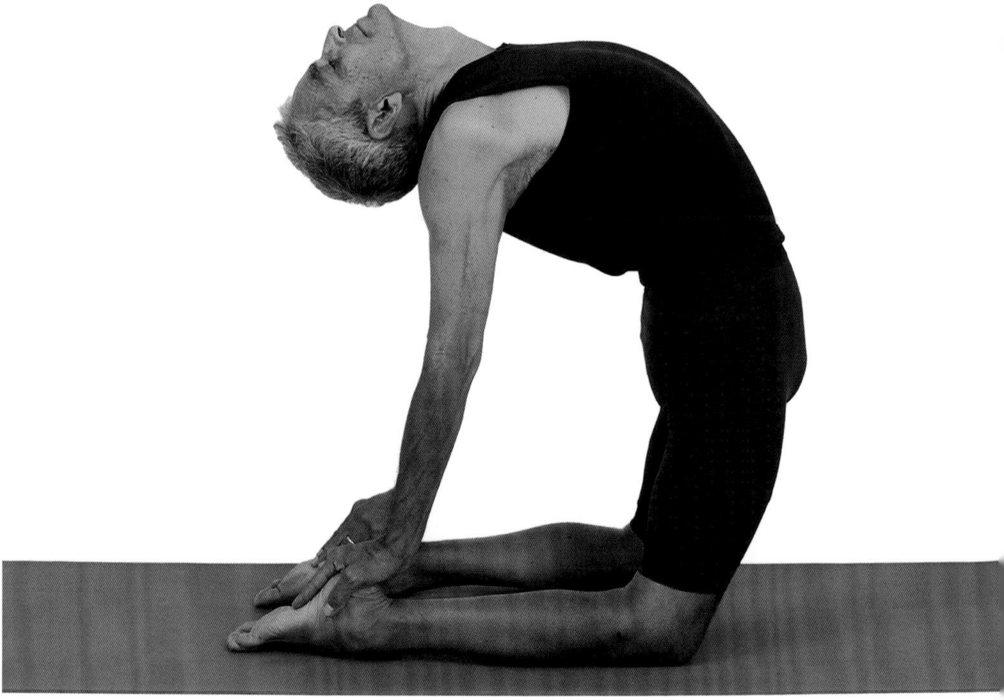

अध्यास्य शेते पदयुग्मव्यस्तं पृष्ठे निधायापि धृतं कराभ्याम् ।
आकुंच्य सम्यग्ध्युदरास्यगधं उष्ट्रश्च पीठं यतयो वदन्ति॥ २:४१ ॥

Adhyāsya śete padayugmavyastam pṛṣṭhe nidhāyāpi dhṛtam karābhyām | ākuñcya samyagdhyudarāsyagaḍham uṣṭraśca pīṭham yatayo vadanti || 2.41 ||

Place the feet down in the "sleeping position" (on the floor) even and separated. Bring the hands to the feet then intensely stretch of the belly. This is called Uṣṭra (camel) seat by the sages. GHERAṆḌA SAMHITA 2:41

## Laghu Vajrāsanam

## लघु वज्रासनम्

**Ekam** - knees hip width, hands on waist, in
**Dwe** - ex, hold ankles, touch top of head to floor
**Nasāgra dṛṣṭi**
**Daśa dīrgha recaka pūraka**
**Trīṇi** - in, come up, ex, utpluthiḥ, in
(transition to next position)
**Catvāri** - ex, caturaṅga daṇḍāsana
**Pañca** - in, ūrdhva mukha śvānāsana
**Ṣat** - ex, adho mukha śvānāsana
**Sapta** - kapotāsana

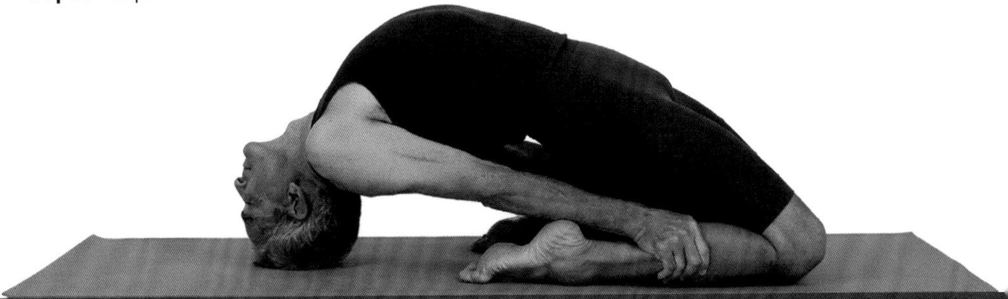

## Kapotāsanam

## कपोतासनम्

**Ekam** - knees hip width, hands on waist, in, lift arms overhead
**Dwe** - ex, arch the back, bring hands to the feet,
hold your feet (heels or ankles), bring elbows to ground
**Nasāgra dṛṣṭi**
**Daśa dīrgha recaka pūraka**
**Trīṇi** - in, come up, ex, utpluthiḥ, in
(transition to next position)
**Catvāri** - ex, caturaṅga daṇḍāsana
**Pañca** - in, ūrdhva mukha śvānāsana
**Ṣat** - ex, adho śvānāsana
**Sapta** - in, daṇḍāsana

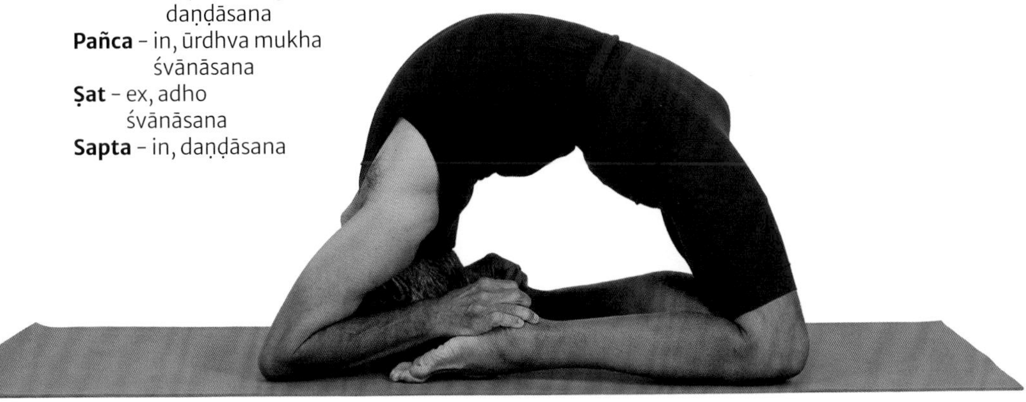

मेरुदण्डग्रन्थिदोर्ढ्यंसंपिपादयिषुः पुमान् ।
कपोतोष्ट्रासनाभ्यासं कुर्यान्मितहियाशनः ॥ योग रहस्य २:२१ ॥

Merudaṇḍagranthidorḍhyamsampipādayiśuḥ pumān |
kapotoṣṭrāsanābhyāsam kuryānmitahiyāśanaḥ || 2.21 ||

For firmness or stability in the spine and grathis (yogic knots of the of the spine) practice Uṣtrāsana and Kapotāsana (3rd deeper variation). Also eat a moderate and suitable diet. YOGA RAHASYA 2:21

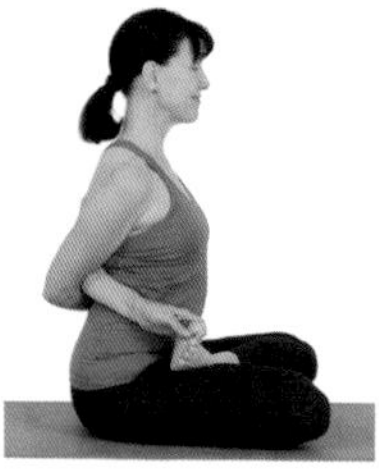

**Baddha padmāsana**
**Ekam** - in, bind feet or hold elbows
**Dwe** - ex, touch top of head to floor, holding feet
**Nasāgra dṛṣṭi**
**Daśa dīrgha recaka pūraka**
**Trīṇi** - in, come up
**Catvāri** - ex, touch head
(repeat trīni/catvāri 3 times)
**Pañca** - ex, touch head
**Nasāgra dṛṣṭi**
**Daśa dīrgha recaka pūraka**
**Ṣat** - in, come up, ex, utpluthiḥ
(transition to next position)
**Sapta** - ex, caturaṅga daṇḍāsana
**Aṣṭau** - in, ūrdhva mukha śvānāsana
**Nava** - ex, adho mukha śvānāsana

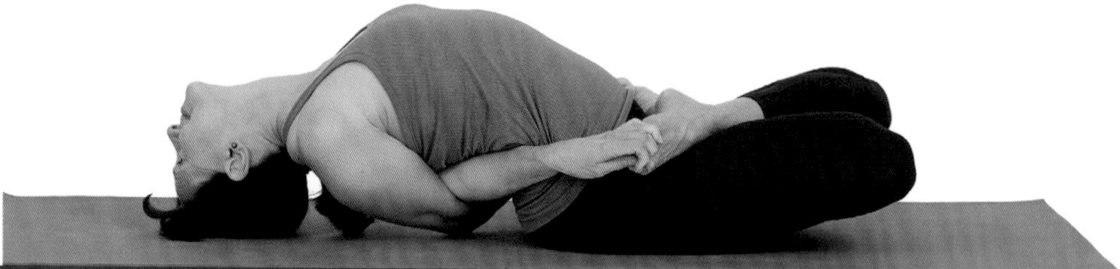

## Prathama Bakāsanam प्रथम बकासनम्

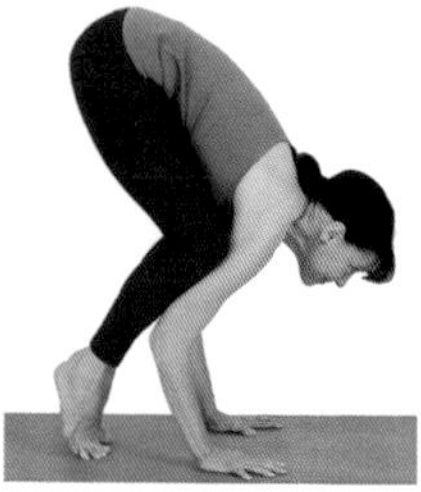

**Ekam** - in, jump feet close to hands, knees to upper arms, ex
**Dwe** - in, come up
**Nasāgra dṛṣṭi**
**Daśa dīrgha recaka pūraka**
(transition to next position)
**Catvāri** - ex, caturaṅga daṇḍāsana
**Pañca** - in, ūrdhva mukha śvānāsana
**Ṣat** - ex, adho mukha śvānāsana

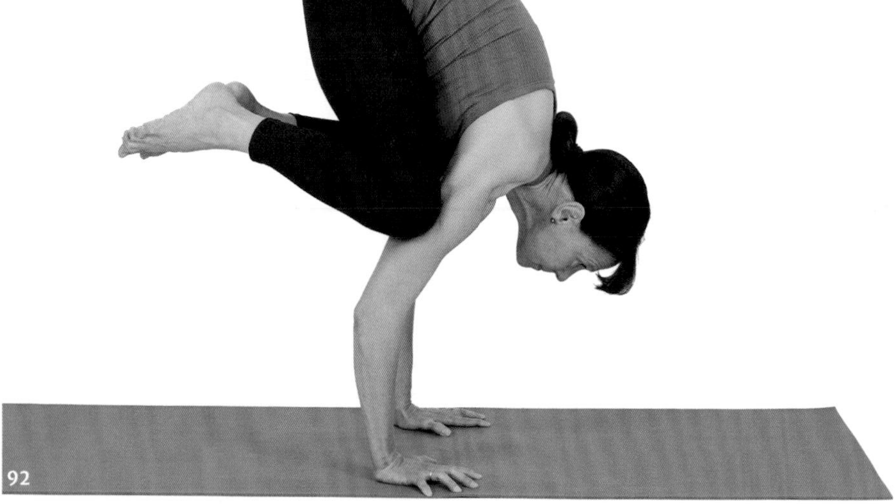

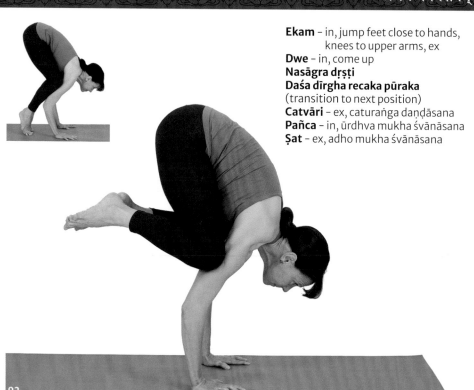

**Sapta** - in, jump into Bakāsana
**Nasāgra dṛṣṭi**
**Daśa dīrgha recaka pūraka**
(transition to next position)
**Catvāri** - ex, caturaṅga daṇḍāsana
**Pañca** - in, ūrdhva mukha śvānāsana
**Ṣat** - ex, adho mukha śvānāsana
**Sapta** - in, daṇḍāsana

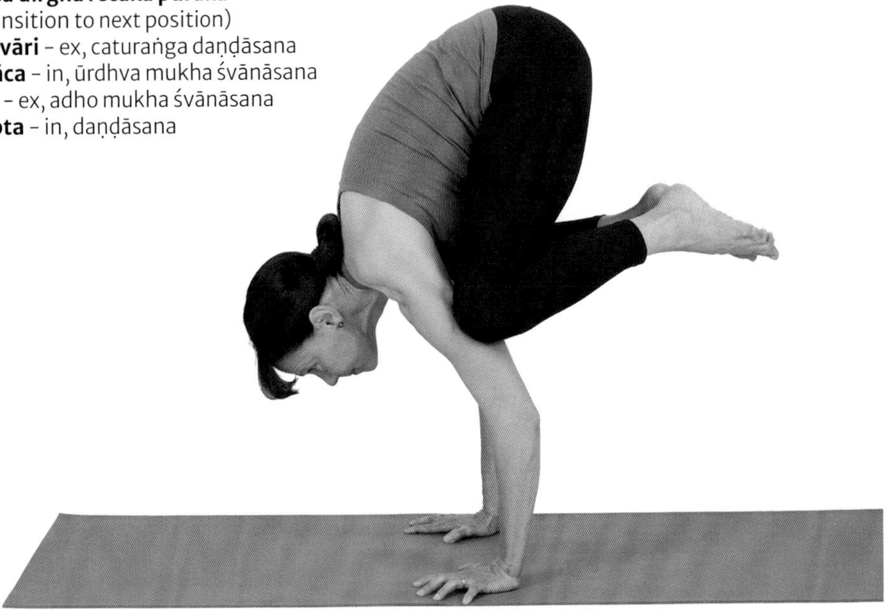

## Bharadvājāsanam भरद्वजासनम्

**Dakṣina bhāga**
**Ekam** - left leg folded, right leg lotus position
**Dwe** - left hand under thigh, right hand bind right leg
**Pārśva dṛṣṭi**
**Daśa dīrgha recaka pūraka**
**Trīṇi** - release, utpluthiḥ
**Catvāri** - ex, caturaṅga daṇḍāsana
**Pañca** - in, ūrdhva mukha śvānāsana
**Ṣat** - ex, adho mukha śvānāsana
**Sapta** - in, daṇḍāsana
**Bharadvājāsana**
**Wama bhāga**
(same as right side - Dakṣina bhāga)
(transition to next position)
**Catvāri** - ex, caturaṅga daṇḍāsana
**Pañca** - in, ūrdhva mukha śvānāsana
**Ṣat** - ex, adho mukha śvānāsana
**Sapta** - in, daṇḍāsana

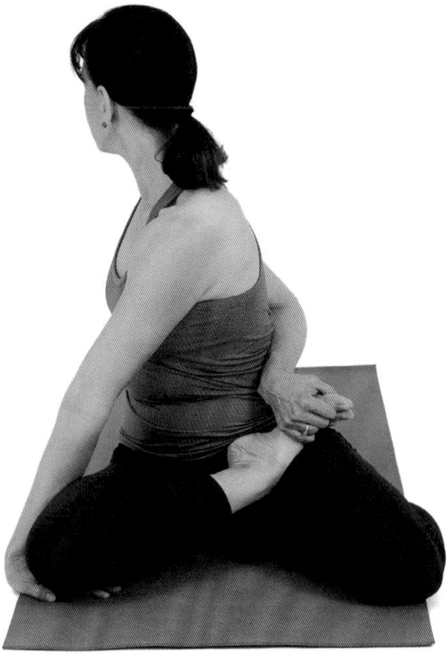

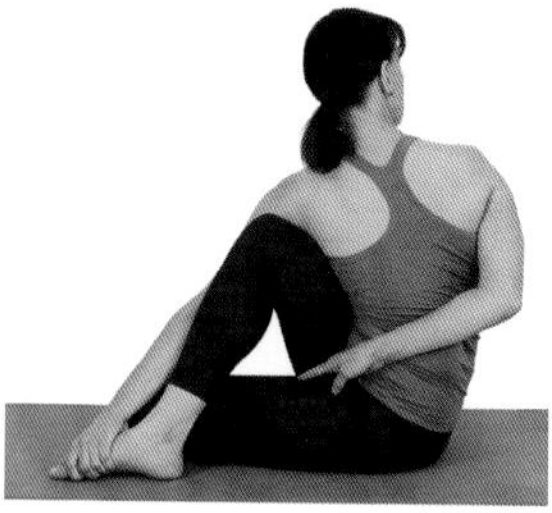

**Dakṣina bhāga**
**Ekam** - left leg folded, right foot to outside of left knee
**Dwe** - left hand hold left foot, right hand to waist
**Pārśva dṛṣṭi**
**Daśa dīrgha recaka pūraka**
**Trīṇi** - release position, utpluthiḥ, in
**Catvāri** - ex, caturaṅga daṇḍāsana
**Pañca** - in, ūrdhva mukha śvānāsana
**Ṣat** - ex, adho mukha śvānāsana
**Sapta** - in, daṇḍāsana
**Ardha Matsyendrāsana**
**Wama bhāga**
(same as right side - Dakṣina bhāga)
(transition to next position)
**Catvāri** - ex, caturaṅga daṇḍāsana
**Pañca** - in, ūrdhva mukha śvānāsana
**Ṣat** - ex, adho mukha śvānāsana
**Sapta** - in, daṇḍāsana, or jumping into right leg ardha bhujapīḍāsana

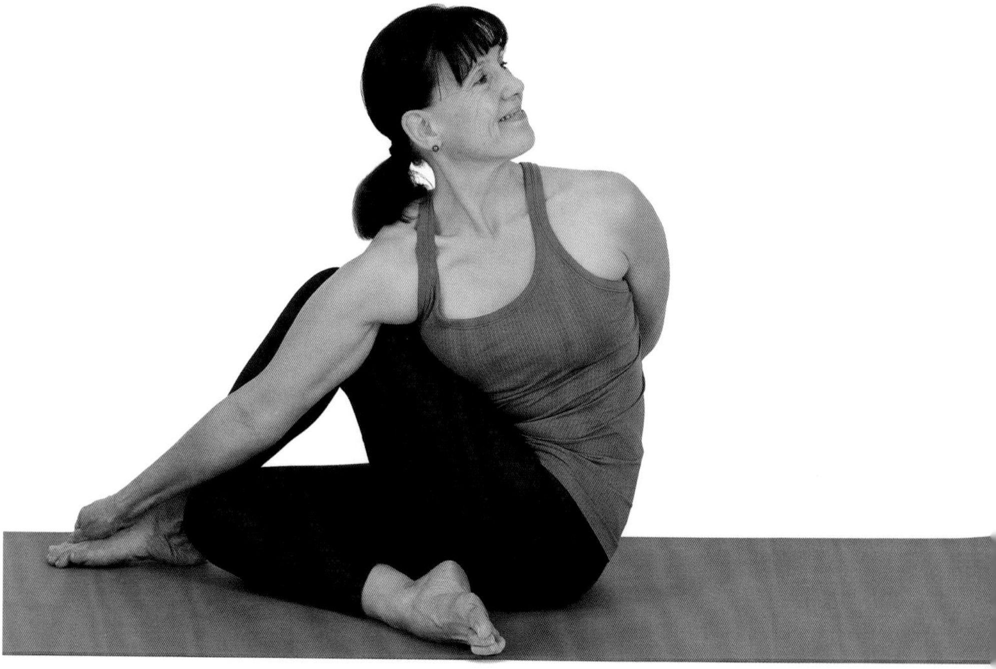

मत्स्येन्द्रपीठां जठरप्रदीप्तं प्रचण्डरुग्मण्डलखन्डनास्त्रं ।
अभ्यास्तः कुण्डलिनीप्रबोधं चन्द्रस्थिरत्वं च ददाति पुम्साम् ॥ १:२७ ॥

Matsyendrapīṭhām jaṭharapradīptam pracaṇḍarugmaṇḍalakhanḍanāstram |
abhyāsataḥ kuṇḍalinīprabodham candra sthiratvam ca dadāti pumsām ||

This asana makes the belly shine and is the weapon to break open the Khaṇḍa circle (abdominal energetic center). Constant practice awakens the kundalini energy (spinal energy) and makes the moon (back of throat) steady. HAṬHA YOGA PRADĪPIKĀ 1:27

**Dakṣina bhāga**
**Ekam** - right leg behind head, in
**Dwe** - ex, forward bend
**Nasāgra dṛṣṭi**
**Daśa dīrgha recaka pūraka**
**Trīṇi** - in, come up, ex, in, utpluthiḥ, in
**Catvāri** - ex, caturaṅga daṇḍāsana
**Pañca** - in, ūrdhva mukha śvānāsana
**Ṣat** - ex, adho mukha śvānāsana
**Sapta** - in, daṇḍāsana (or ardha bhujapīḍāsana)
**Eka Pāda Śīrṣāsana**
**Wama bhāga**
(same as right side - Dakṣina bhāga)
(transition to next position)
**Catvāri** - ex, caturaṅga daṇḍāsana
**Pañca** - in, ūrdhva mukha śvānāsana
**Ṣat** - ex, adho mukha śvānāsana
**Sapta** - dwi pāda śīrṣāsana

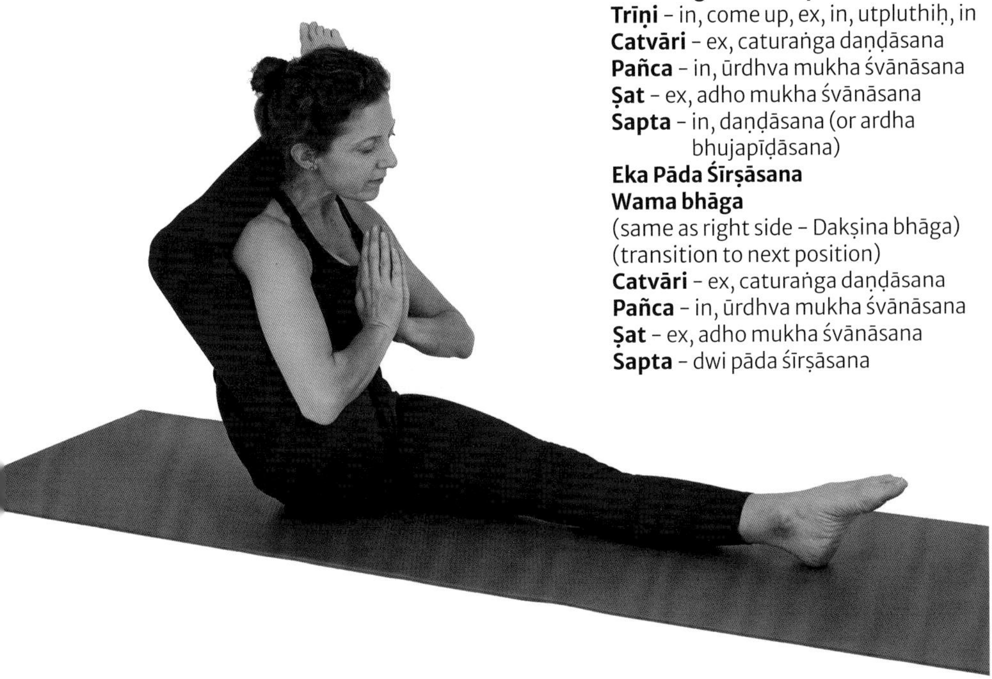

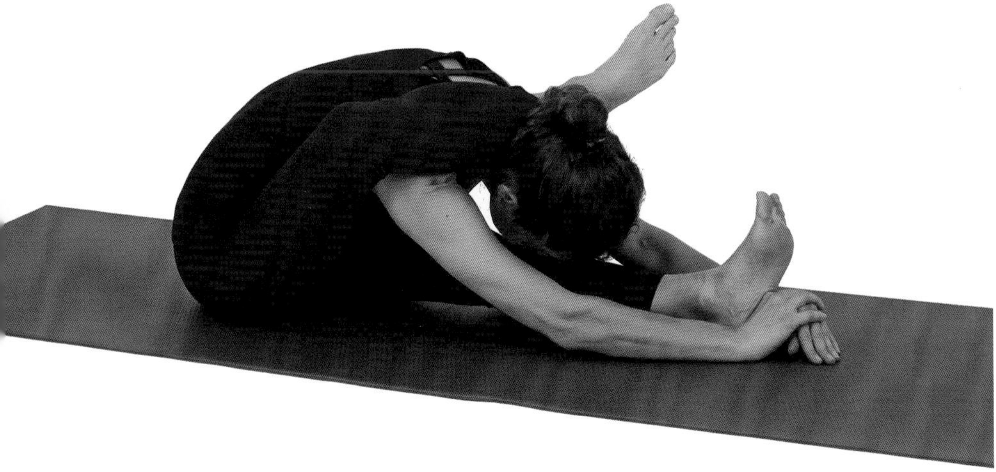

**Dakṣina bhāga**
**Ekam** - in, bhujapīḍāsana position
**Dwe** - ex, legs behind head, alternate left leg then right behind, palms together
**Nasāgra dṛṣṭi**
**Daśa dīrgha recaka pūraka**
**Trīṇi** - utpluthiḥ, in
**Nasāgra dṛṣṭi**
**Daśa dīrgha recaka pūraka**
(transition to next position)
**Catvāri** - ex, caturaṅga daṇḍāsana
**Pañca** - in, ūrdhva mukha śvānāsana

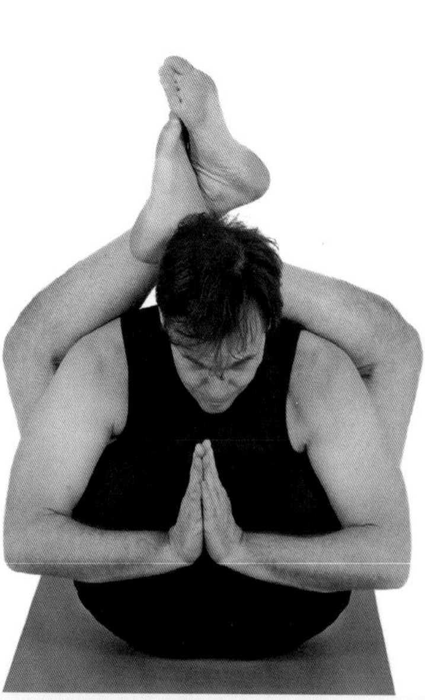

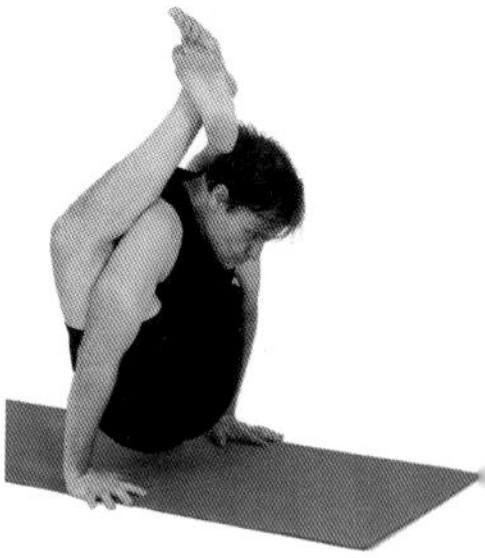

कण्ठपृष्ठे क्षिपेत्पादौ पाशवत् दृढबन्धनम् ।
सैव स्यात् पाशिनी मुद्रा शक्ति प्रबोध कारिणी ॥ ३:६५ ॥

Kaṇṭhapṛṣṭhe kṣipetpādau pāśavat dṛḍhabandhanam |
saiva syāt pāśinīmudrā śakti prabodha kāriṇī || 3:65 ||

Place the legs at the back of the throat (behind the neck), tied and bound firmly. Indeed this is Pāshinī Mudra, which when practiced awakens the Śakti (internal energy of the body).

GHERAṆḌA SAMHITA 3:65

## Yoga Nidrāsanam    योग निद्रासनम्

**Ekam** - ex, samasthitiḥ (laying down)
**Dwe** - feet behind head, right leg behind left leg, bind hands behind back
**Nasāgra dṛṣṭi**
**Daśa dīrgha recaka pūraka**
**Trīṇi** - release position, cakrāsana, in
(transition to next position)
**Catvāri** - ex, caturaṅga daṇḍāsana
**Pañca** - in, ūrdhva mukha śvānāsana
**Ṣat** - ex, adho mukha śvānāsana
**Sapta** - titibhāsana

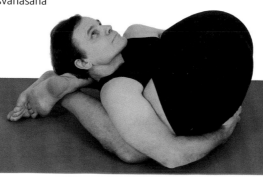

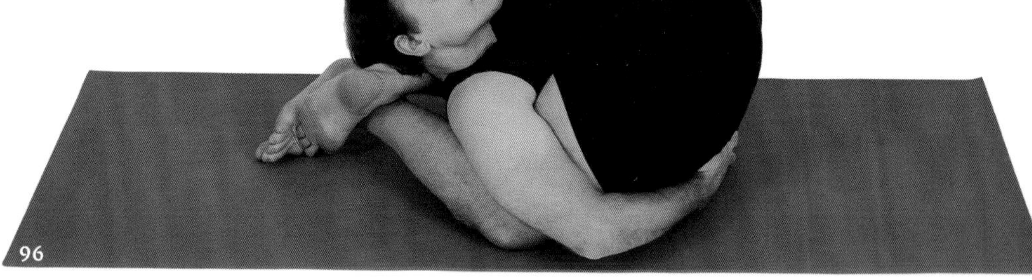

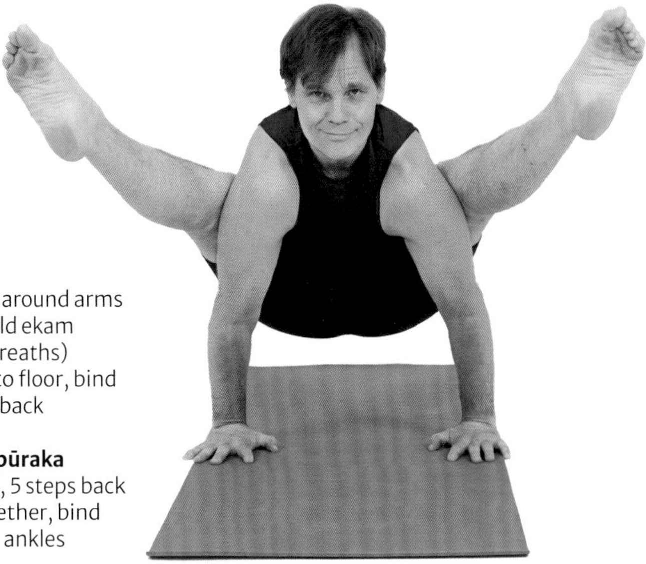

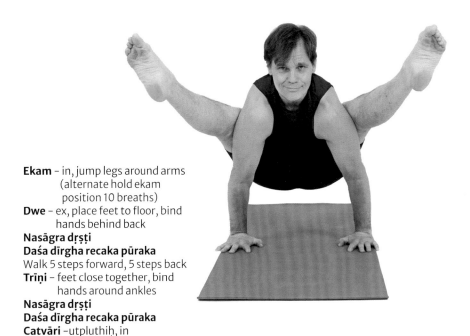

**Ekam** - in, jump legs around arms (alternate hold ekam position 10 breaths)
**Dwe** - ex, place feet to floor, bind hands behind back
**Nasāgra dṛṣṭi**
**Daśa dīrgha recaka pūraka**
Walk 5 steps forward, 5 steps back
**Trīṇi** - feet close together, bind hands around ankles
**Nasāgra dṛṣṭi**
**Daśa dīrgha recaka pūraka**
**Catvāri** -utpluthiḥ, in (transition to next position)
**Pañca** - ex, caturaṅga daṇḍāsana
**Ṣat** - in, ūrdhva mukha śvānāsana
**Sapta** - ex, adho mukha śvānāsana

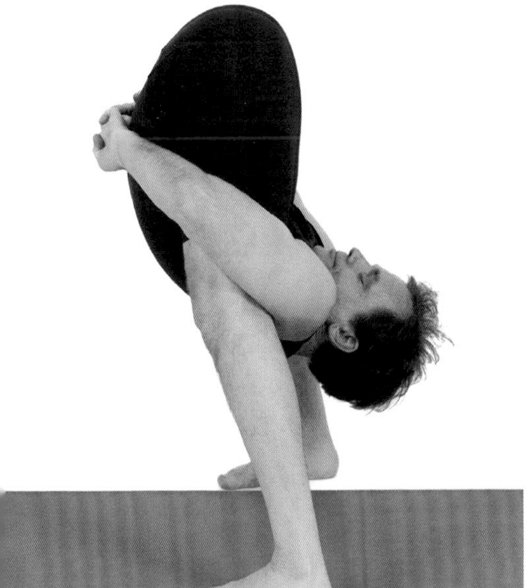

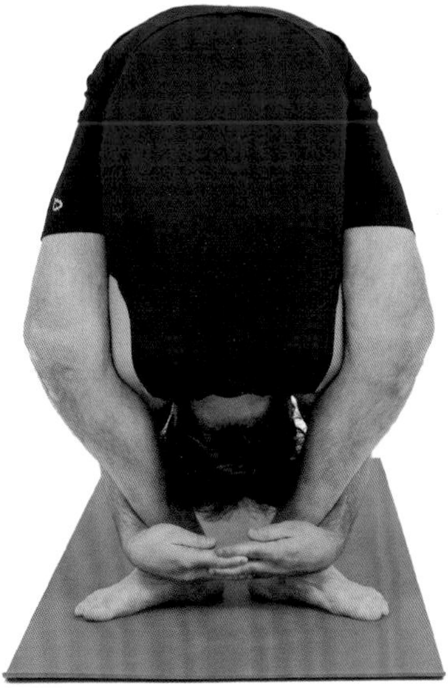

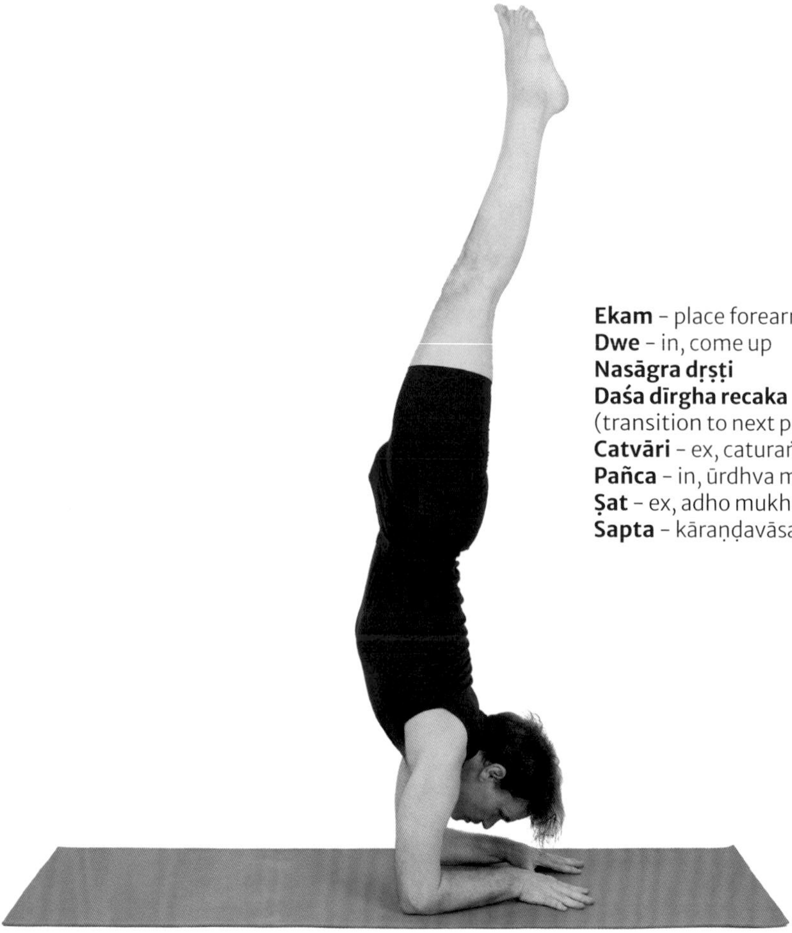

**Ekam** – place forearms to ground
**Dwe** – in, come up
**Nasāgra dṛṣṭi**
**Daśa dīrgha recaka pūraka**
(transition to next position)
**Catvāri** – ex, caturaṅga daṇḍāsana
**Pañca** – in, ūrdhva mukha śvānāsana
**Ṣat** – ex, adho mukha śvānāsana
**Sapta** – kāraṇḍavāsana

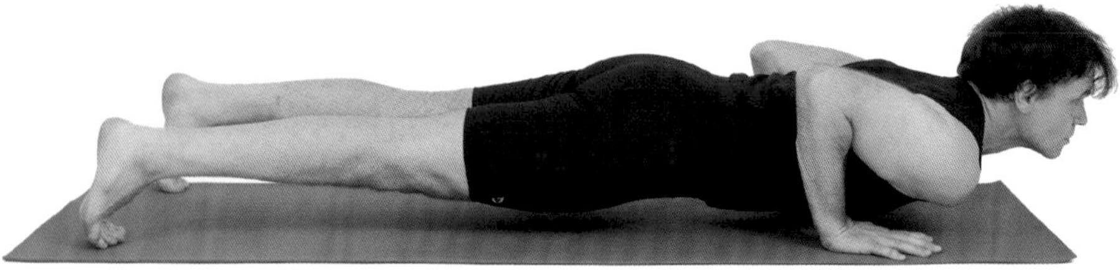

**Ekam** - ex, place forearms to ground
**Dwe** - in, come up to piccha mayūrāsana
**Trīṇi** - ex, legs into padmāsana, in
**Catvāri** - ex, kāraṇḍavāsana, knees on upper arms
**Nasāgra dṛṣṭi**
**Daśa dīrgha recaka pūraka**
**Pañca** - in, come up
**Ṣat** - ex, feet to head
**Vṛścikāsana**
**Nasāgra dṛṣṭi**
**Daśa dīrgha recaka pūraka**
**Sapta** - in, piccha mayūrāsana
**Aṣṭau** - ex, caturaṅga daṇḍāsana (transition to next position)
**Nava** - in, ūrdhva mukha śvānāsana
**Daśa** - ex, adho mukha śvānāsana
**Ekādaśa** - in, feet to hands
**Dvādaśa** - ex, heads to knees
**Trayodaśa** - in, arms up, ex, samasthitiḥ

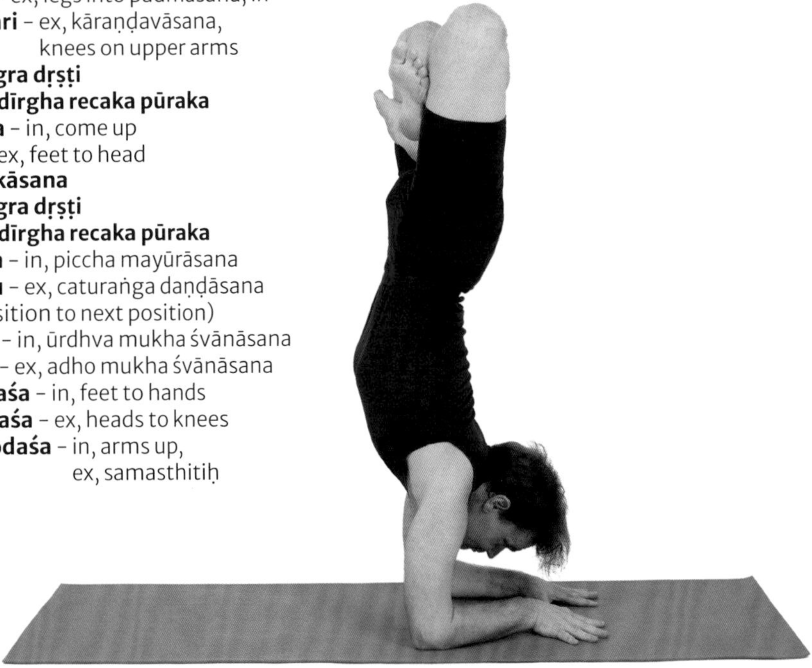

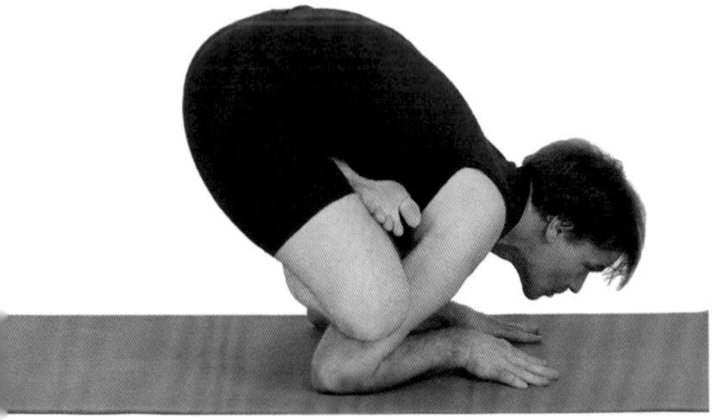

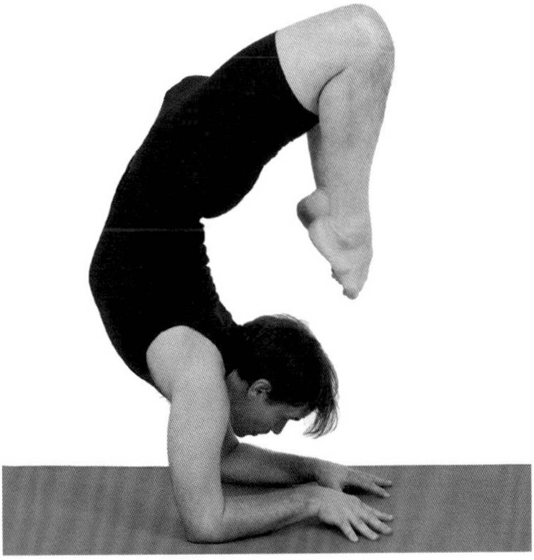

सप्तचक्र क्षालनाय
वृश्चिकासन विशेषकान् ॥ २:२० ॥

Saptacakrakṣālanāya vṛścikāsanaviśeṣakān || 2:20 ||

Scorpion positions have the special property of cleaning the seven chakras. YOGA RAHASYA 2:20

**Ekam** – jump feet apart, place hands facing backward between feet, in, head up
**Dwe** – ex, head down
**Trīṇi** – in, head up
**Catvāri** – jump back, elbows to abdomen close to navel, balance on elbows
**Nasāgra dṛṣṭi**
**Daśa dīrgha reckaka pūraka**

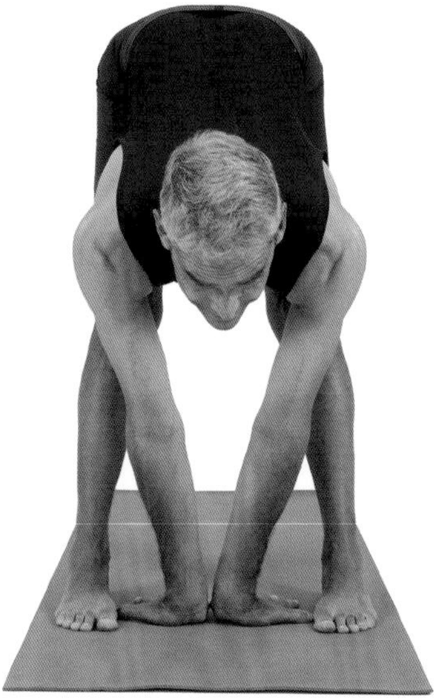

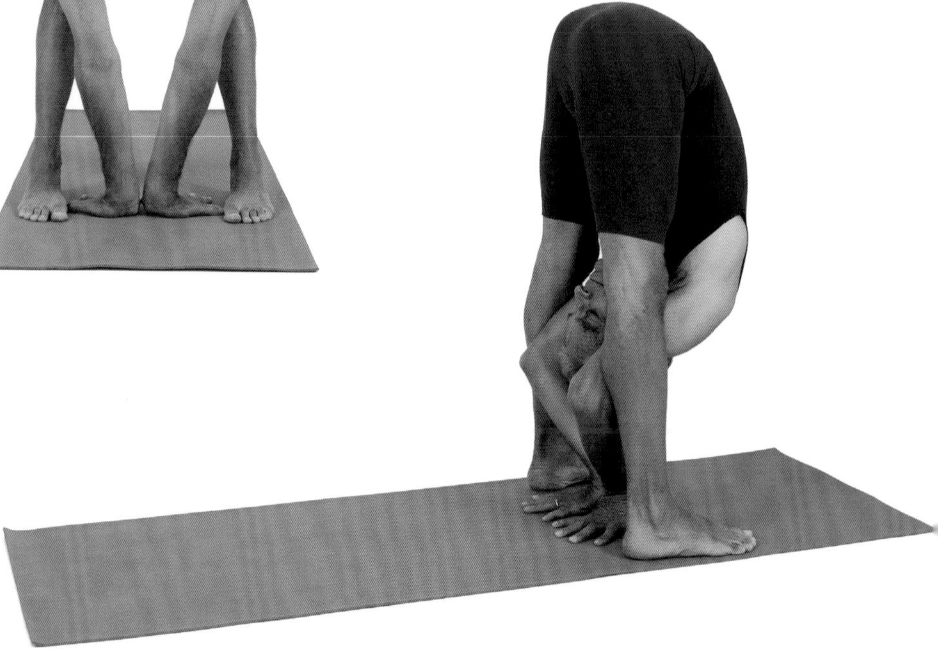

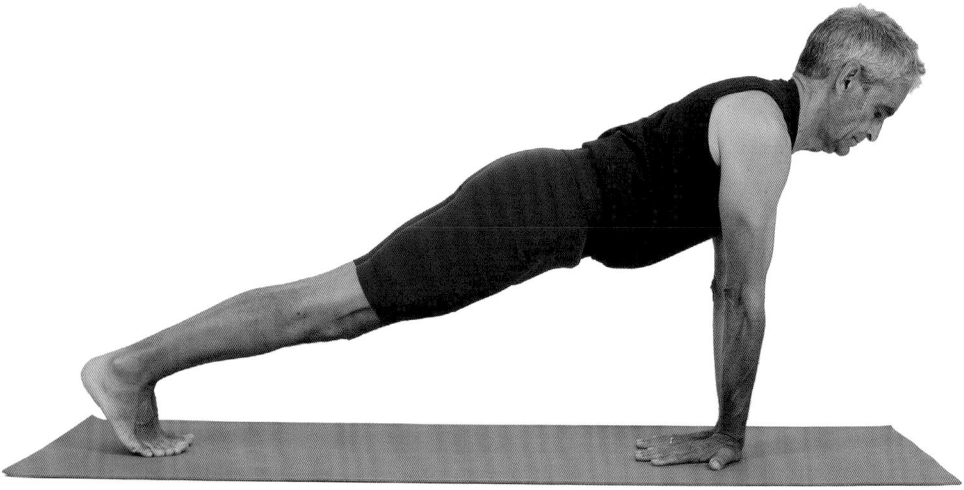

(transition to next position)
**Pañca** - in, ūrdhva mukha śvānāsana
**Ṣat** - ex, adho mukha śvānāsana
**Sapta** - in, jump around feet hands head up
**Aṣṭau** - ex, head down
**Nava** - in, head up, ex, samasthitiḥ

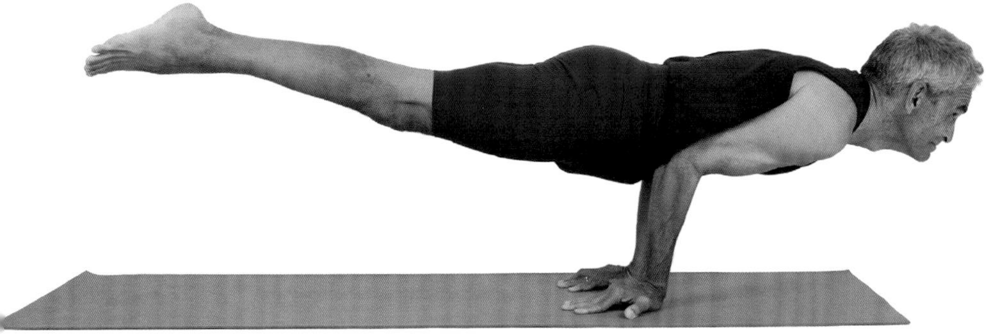

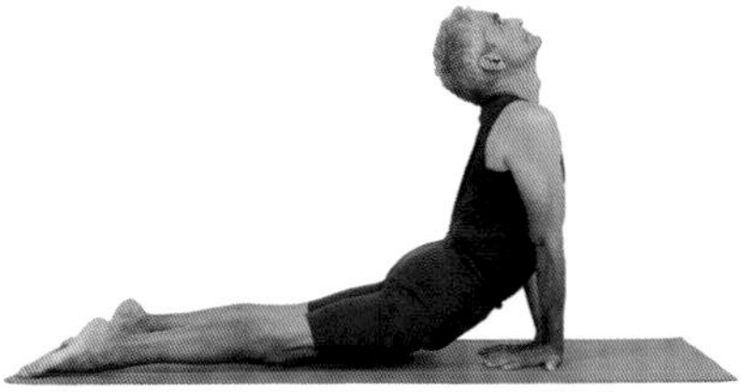

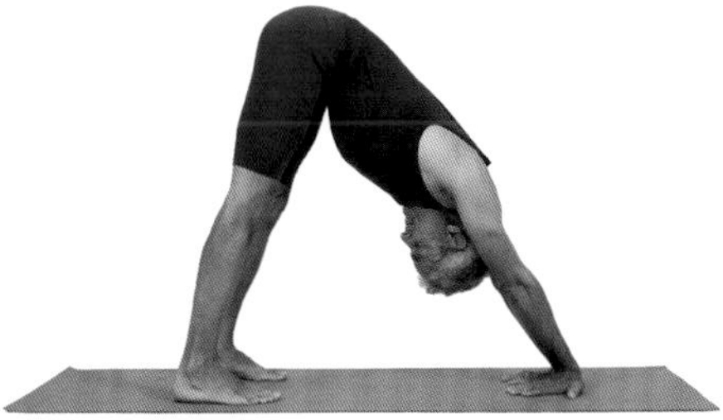

हरति सकलोगानाशुगुल्मोदरादीनभिभवति च दोषानासानं श्रीमयूरम् ।
बहु कदशनभुक्तं भस्म कुर्यादशेषं जनयति जठराग्निं जारयेत्कालकूटम् ॥ १:३२ ॥

Harati sakalogānāśugulmodarādīnabhibhavati ca doṣānāsām śrīmayūram |
bahu kadashanabhuktam bhasma kuryādaśeṣam janayati jaṭharāgnim jārayetkālakūṭam ||

This (asana) takes away all diseases particularly chronic enlargement of the spleen and enlargement of the stomach. It makes the belly shine clarifying the the Dośa (our Ayurvedic constitution). This great Mayūram turns to ashes the bad or remaining food (i.e., constipation), destroys the deadly poison Hālāhala, and secures the digestive fire. HAṬHA YOGA PRADĪPIKĀ 1:30

**Prathama sūrya namaskāraḥ**
**Ekam** – in, arms up
**Dwe** – ex, head down
**Trīṇi** – in, head up
**Catvāri** – ex, caturaṅga daṇḍāsana
Jump 5 times forward and back
**Pañca** – in, ūrdhva mukha śvānāsana
**Ṣat** – adho mukha śvānāsana
**Sapta** – in, feet between hands, head up
**Aṣṭau** – ex, head down
**Nava** – in, come up
**Samasthitiḥ**

Optional Counting
(transition to next position)
**Pañca** – in, ūrdhva mukha śvānāsana
**Ṣat** – adho mukha śvānāsana
**Sapta** – daṇḍāsana

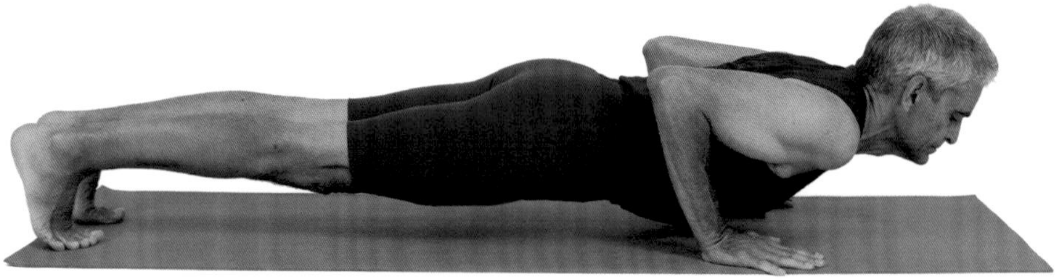

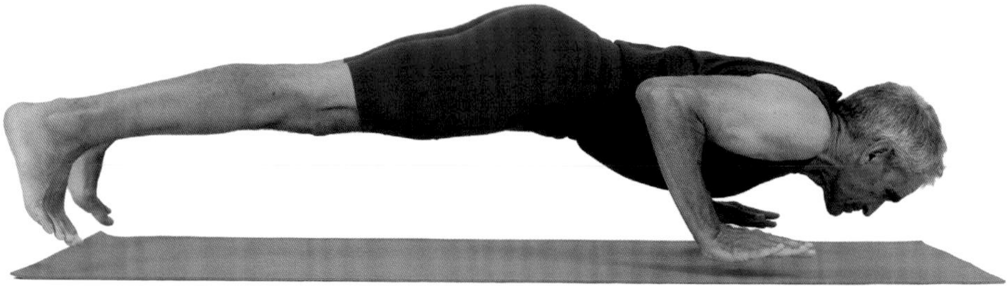

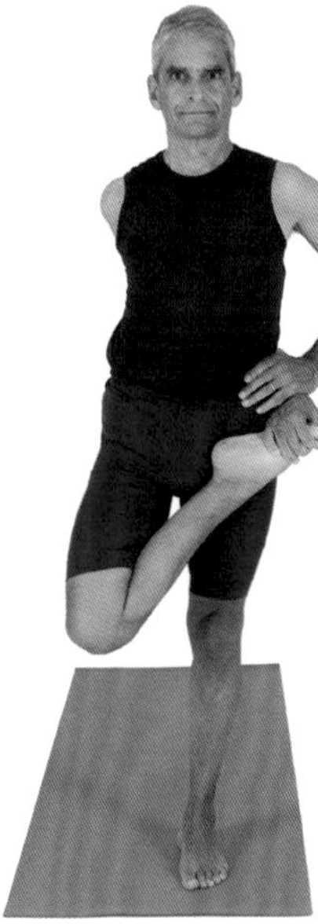

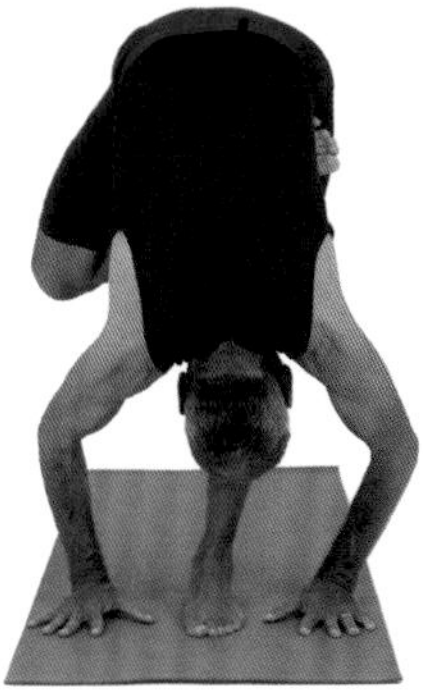

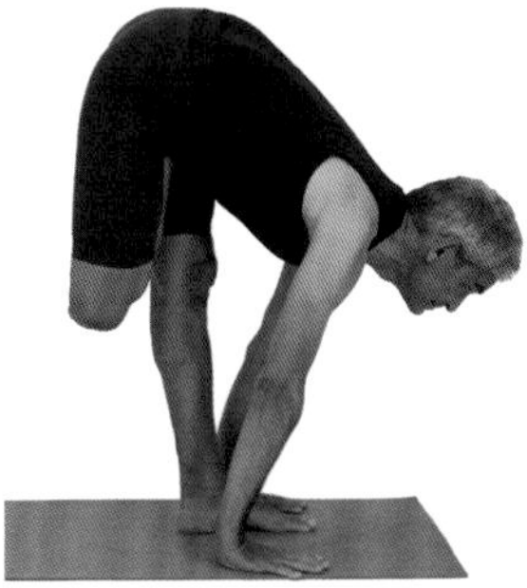

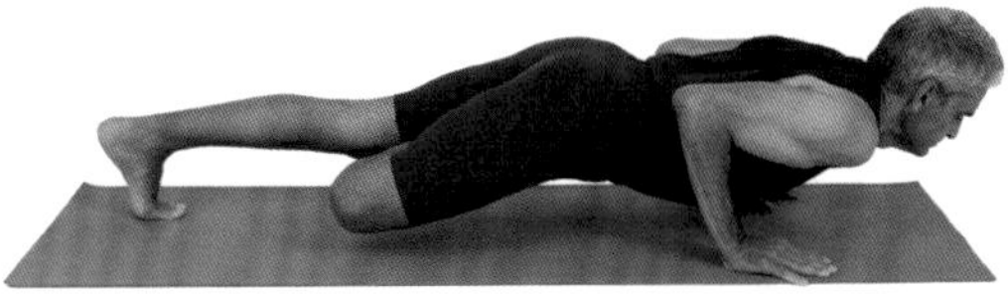

**Ekam** - right leg ardha padmasāsana, bind foot, in
**Dwe** - ex, both hands to the floor
**Trīṇi** - in, head up
**Catvāri** - ex, caturaṅga daṇḍāsana, right leg ardha padmāsana
**Pañca** - in, ūrdhva mukha śvānāsana, right leg ardha padmāsana
**Ṣat** - ex, adho mukha śvānāsana, right leg ardha padmāsana
**Sapta** - jump right knee, place next to ankle or on middle calf area, cross elbows, right on top, join palms
**Dakṣina bhāga**
**Hastāgra dṛṣṭi**
**Daśa dīrgha recaka pūraka**
(utpluthiḥ, in)
**Catvāri** - ex, caturaṅga daṇḍāsana, right leg ardha padmāsana
**Pañca** - in, ūrdhva mukha śvānāsana, right leg ardha padmāsana
**Ṣat** - ex, adho mukha śvānāsana, right leg ardha padmāsana

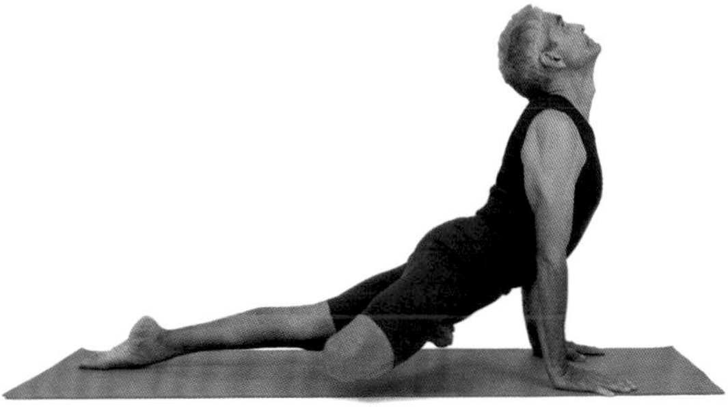

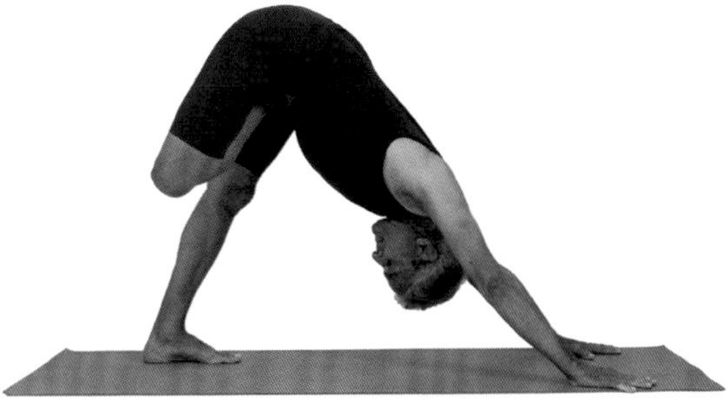

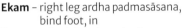

**Vatayanāsana**
**Wama bhāga**
(change legs, left ardha padmāsana)
**Sapta** - jump left knee in, place next to ankle or on middle calf area, cross elbows, left on top, join palms
**Hastāgra dṛṣṭi**
**Daśa dīrgha recaka pūraka**
(same as right side - Dakṣina bhāga)
(transition to next position)
**Catvāri** - ex, caturaṅga daṇḍāsana, left ardha padmāsana
**Pañca** - in, ūrdhva mukha śvānāsana, left ardha padmāsana
**Ṣat** - ex, adho mukha śvānāsana, left ardha padmāsana
**Sapta** - in, right foot between hands, bind left ardha padmāsana
**Aṣṭau** - ex, head down
**Nava** - in, head up, ex, come up with foot in ardha padmāsana
**Samasthitiḥ**

Optional Counting
(transition into Parighasana after left side)
**Catvāri** - ex, caturaṅga daṇḍāsana, left ardha padmāsana
**Pañca** - in, ūrdhva mukha śvānāsana, left ardha padmāsana
**Ṣat** - ex, adho mukha śvānāsana, both feet on the mat, in daṇḍāsana

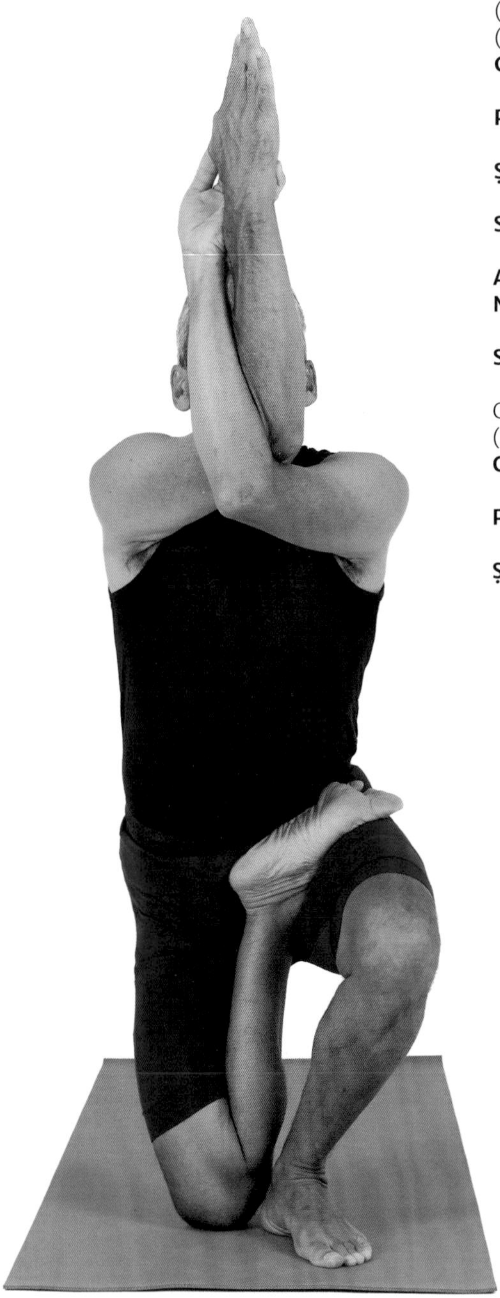

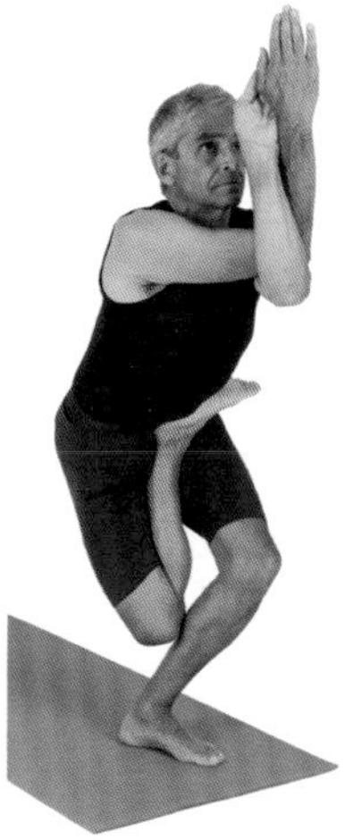

**Prathama sūrya namaskāraḥ**
**Ekam** - in, hands up
**Dwe** - ex, head down
**Trīṇi** - in, head up
**Catvāri** - ex, caturaṅga daṇḍāsana
**Pañca** - in, ūrdhva mukha śvānāsana
**Ṣat** - ex, adho mukha śvānāsana
**Sapta** - in, daṇḍāsana
**Dakṣina bhāga**
**Ekam** - right leg folded, left leg to the side, hands to waist, in
**Dwe** - ex, hold left foot
**Ūrdhva dṛṣṭi**
**Daśa dīrgha recaka pūraka**
**Trīṇi** - in, come up, ex, utpluthiḥ, in
**Catvāri** - ex, caturaṅga daṇḍāsana
**Pañca** - in, ūrdhva mukha śvānāsana
**Ṣat** - ex, adho mukha śvānāsana
**Sapta** - in, daṇḍāsana
**Parighāsana**
**Wama bhāga**
(same as right side - Dakṣina bhāga)
(transition to next posture)
**Trīṇi** - in, come up, ex, utpluthiḥ, in
**Catvāri** - ex, caturaṅga daṇḍāsana
**Pañca** - in, ūrdhva mukha śvānāsana
**Ṣat** - ex, adho mukha śvānāsana
**Sapta** - in, daṇḍāsana

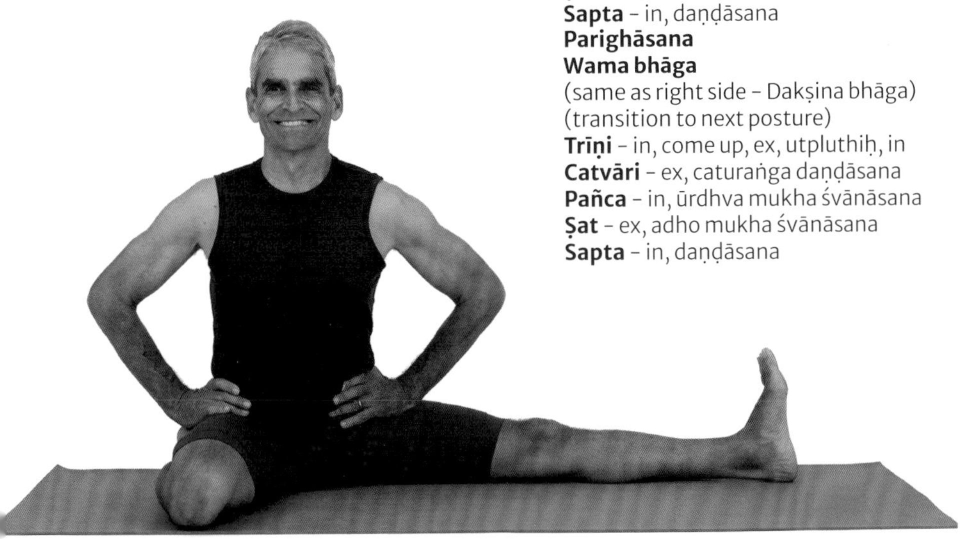

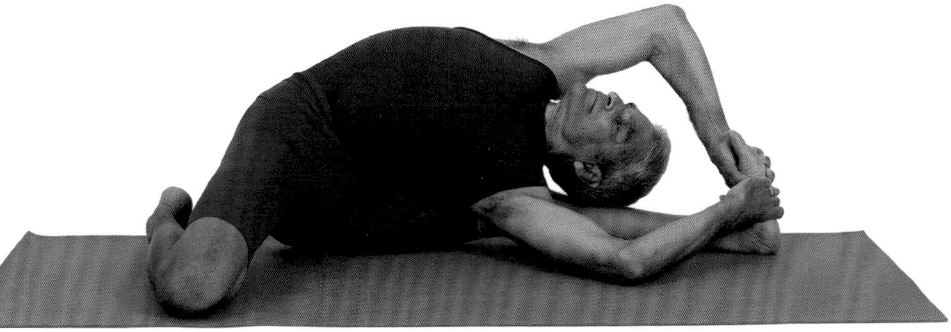

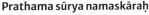

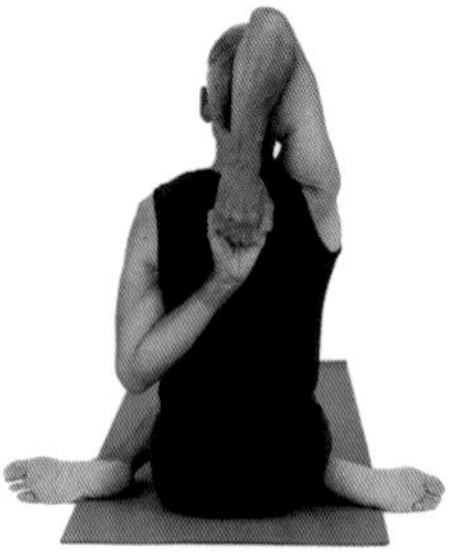

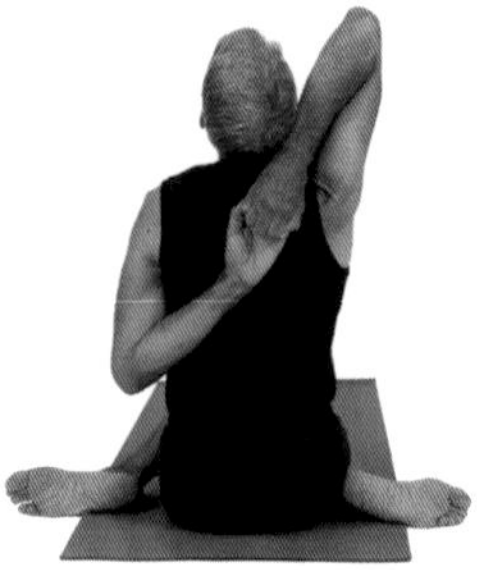

**Dakṣina bhāga**
**Ekam** - fold left leg to right hip, then right leg to left hip, heels close together (alternate, hips on floor ankles to the sides of body)
**Dwe** - right arm over right shoulder, bind with left hand behind back
**Ūrdhva dṛṣṭi**
**Daśa dīrgha recaka pūraka**
**Trīṇi** - release, in, utplitihiḥ
**Catvāri** - ex, caturaṅga daṇḍāsana
**Pañca** - in, ūrdhva mukha śvānāsana
**Ṣat** - ex, adho mukha śvānāsana
**Sapta** - daṇḍāsana
**Gomukhāsana**
**Wama bhāga**
(same as right side - Dakṣina bhāga)

Optional Counting
**Dakṣina bhāga**
**Ekam** - fold left leg to right hip, then right leg to left hip, heels close together, hold the front knee, fingers interlaced
**Nasāgra dṛṣṭi**
**Daśa dīrgha reckaka pūraka**
**Dwe** - right arm over right shoulder bind with left hand behind back
**Ūrdhva dṛṣṭi**
**Daśa dīrgha recaka pūraka**
**Trīṇi** - release, in, utplitihiḥ

(transition to next posture)
**Catvāri** - ex, caturaṅga daṇḍāsana
**Pañca** - in, ūrdhva mukha śvānāsana
**Ṣat** - ex, adho mukha śvānāsana
**Sapta** - daṇḍāsana

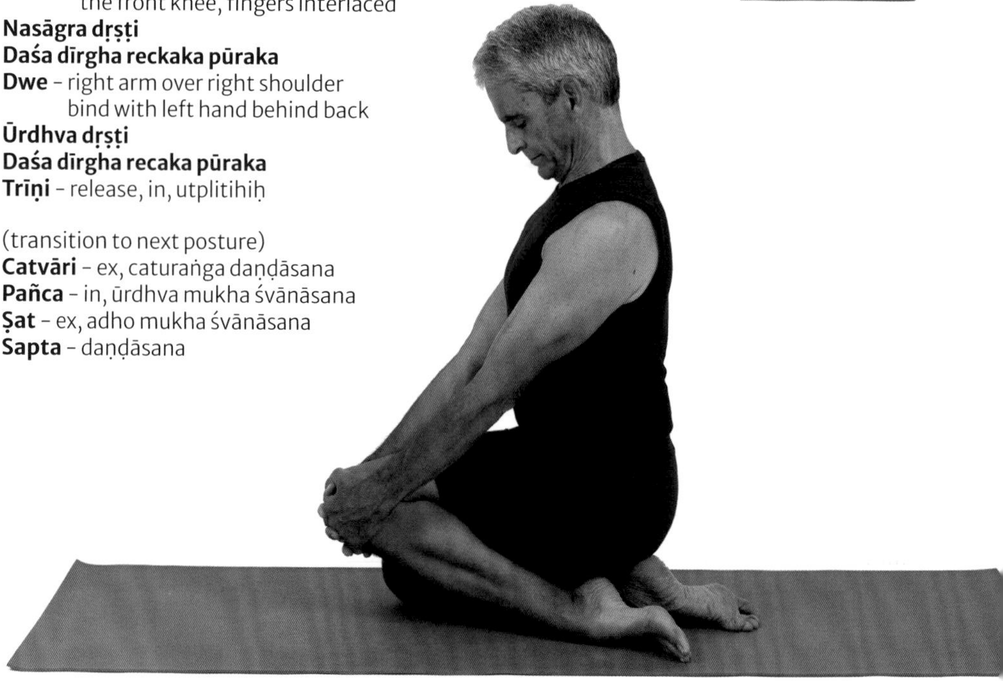

सव्ये दक्षिणगुल्फं तु पृष्ठपार्श्वे नियोजयेत् ।
दक्षिणे तथा सव्यं गोमुखं गोमुखाकृति ॥ १:२० ॥

Savye dakṣiṇagulpham tu pṛṣṭhapārśve niyojayet |
dakṣine tathā savyam gomukham gomukhākṛti || 1:20 ||

Indeed at the side (hip), joined to the back, place the right ankle. Now the left (ankle) on the right side. This is the Gomukha (āsana) the cow-face form. HAṬHA YOGA PRADĪPIKĀ 1:20

**Dakṣina bhāga**
**Samasthitiḥ** (laying down)
**Ekam** - halāsana position, right leg lotus position, bind foot
**Nasāgra dṛṣṭi**
**Daśa dīrgha recaka pūraka**

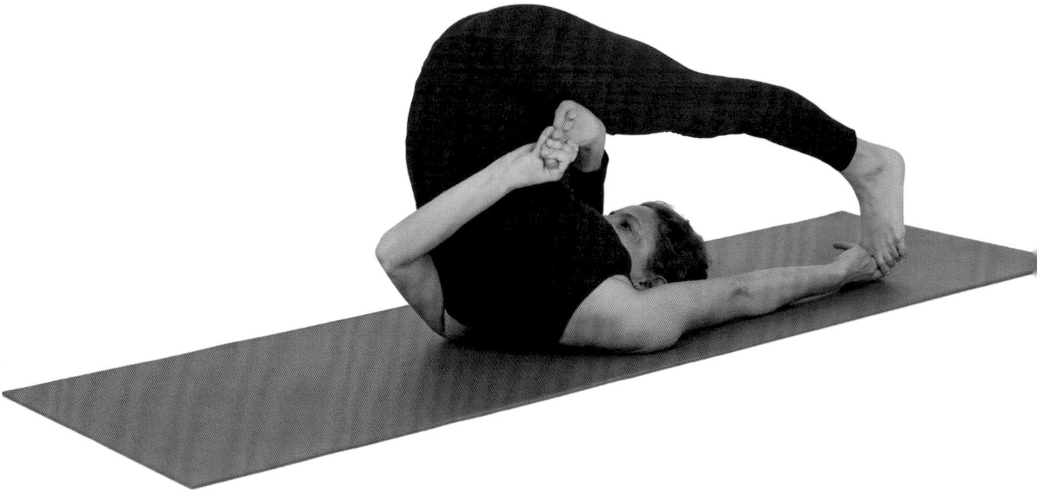

**Dwe** - roll up into bharadvājāsana
**Nasāgra dṛṣṭi**
**Daśa dīrgha recaka pūraka**
**Trīṇi** - release, utplitihiḥ, in
**Catvāri** ex, caturaṅga daṇḍāsana
**Pañca** - in, ūrdhva mukha śvānāsana
**Ṣat** - ex, adho mukha śvānāsana
**Sapta** - daṇḍāsana
**Supta** ūrdhva pāda vajrāsana
**Wama bhāga**
(same as right side - Dakṣina bhāga)
(transition to next posture)
**Catvāri** - ex, caturaṅga daṇḍāsana
**Pañca** - in, ūrdhva mukha śvānāsana
**Ṣat** - ex, adho mukha śvānāsana
**Sapta** - mukta hasta śīrshāsana

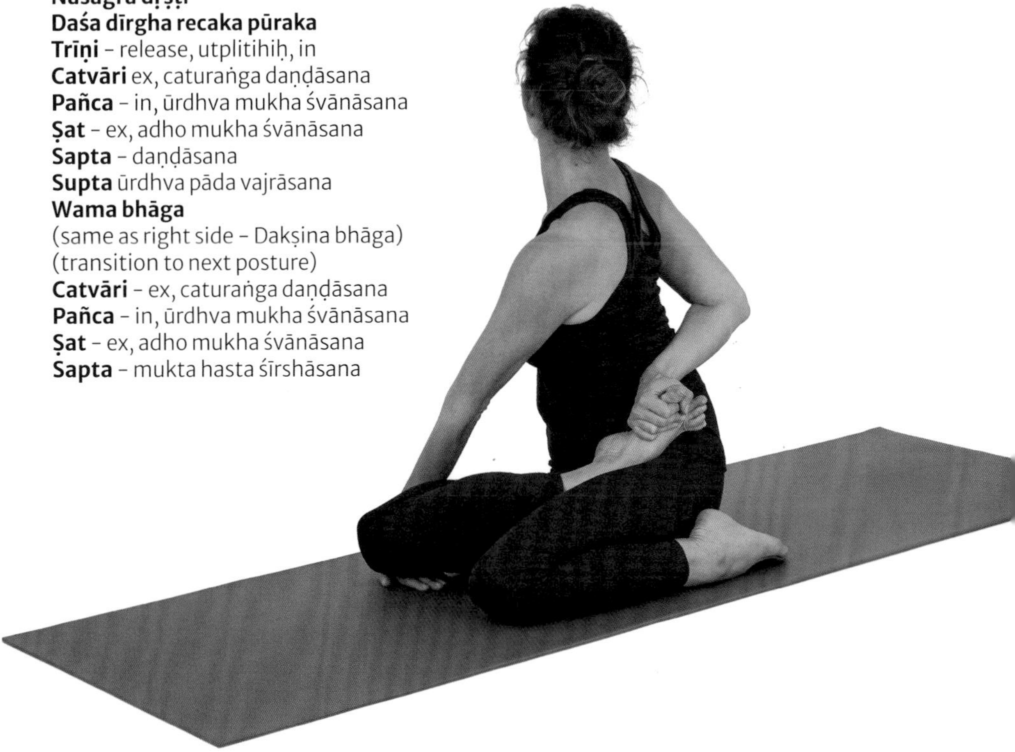

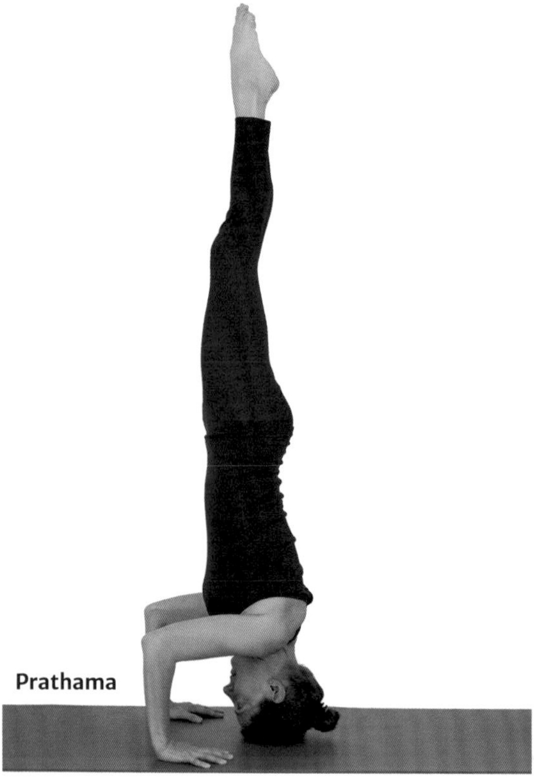

Prathama

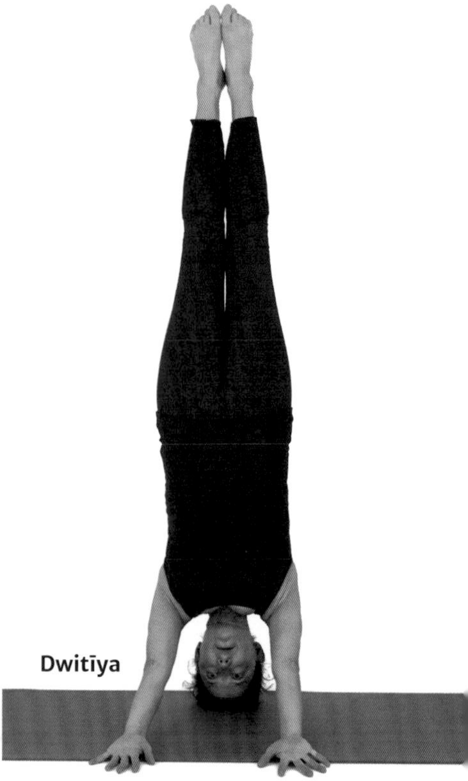

Dwitīya

**Ekam** - place head and hands
**Dwe** - in, come up
**Nasāgra dṛṣṭi**
**Daśa dīrgha recaka pūraka**
**Catvāri** - ex, caturaṅga daṇḍāsana
**Pañca** - in, ūrdhva mukha śvānāsana
**Ṣat** - ex, adho mukha śvānāsana
(repeat ekam to ṣat for all of the headstands)

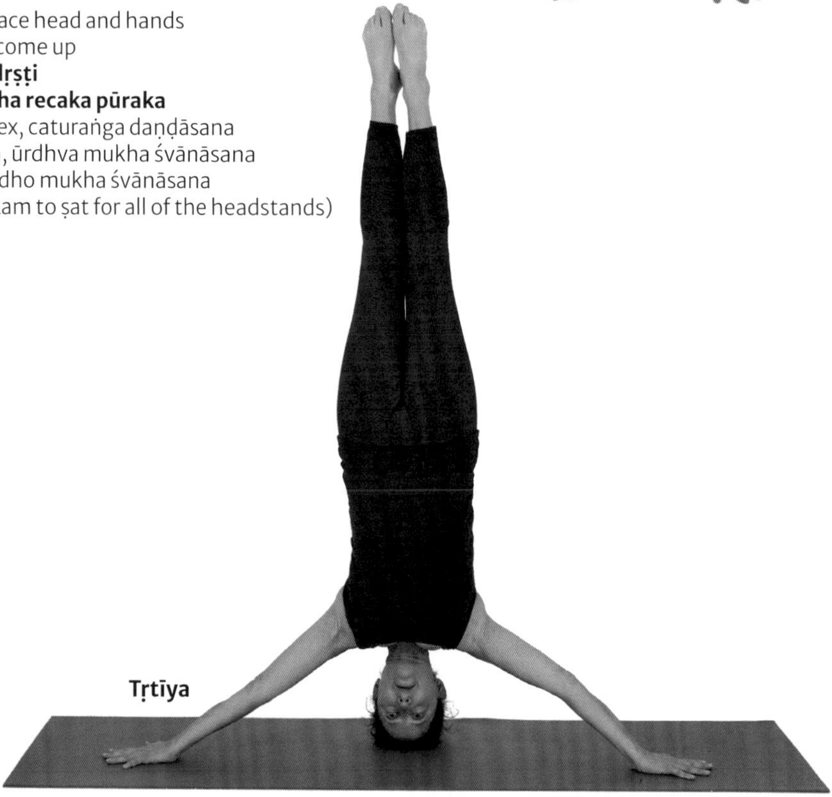

Tṛtīya

**Ekam** - place head and hands
**Dwe** - in, come up
**Nasāgra dṛṣṭi**
**Daśa dīrgha recaka pūraka**
**Catvāri** - ex, caturaṅga daṇḍāsana
**Pañca** - in, ūrdhva mukha śvānāsana
**Ṣat** - ex, adho mukha śvānāsana
(repeat ekam to ṣat for all of the headstands)

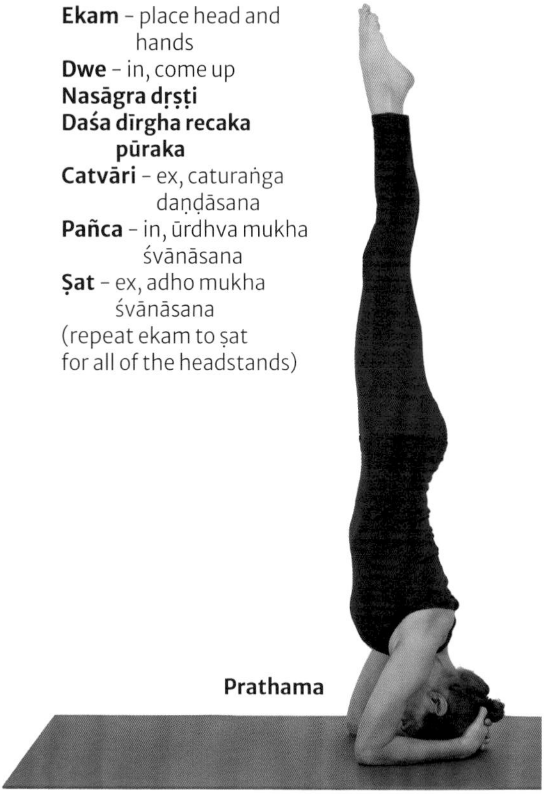
**Prathama**

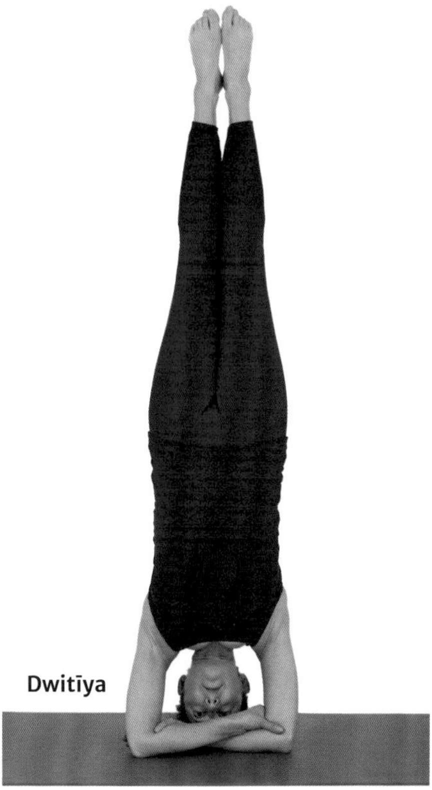
**Dwitīya**

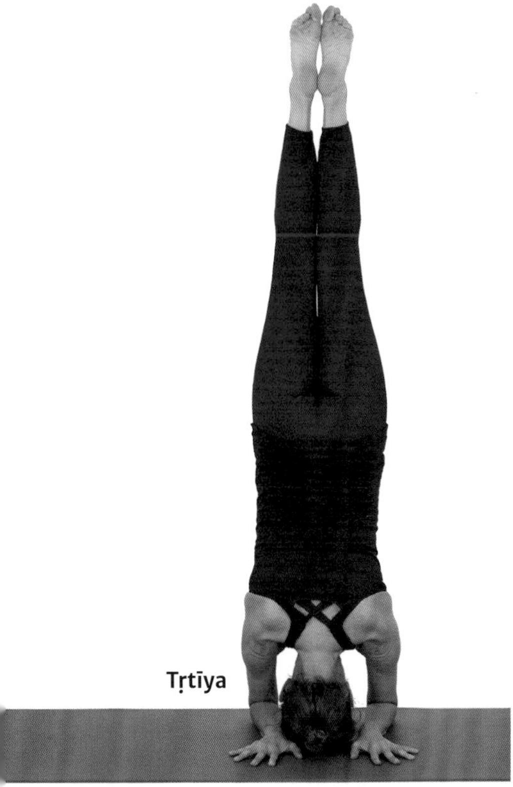
**Tṛtīya**

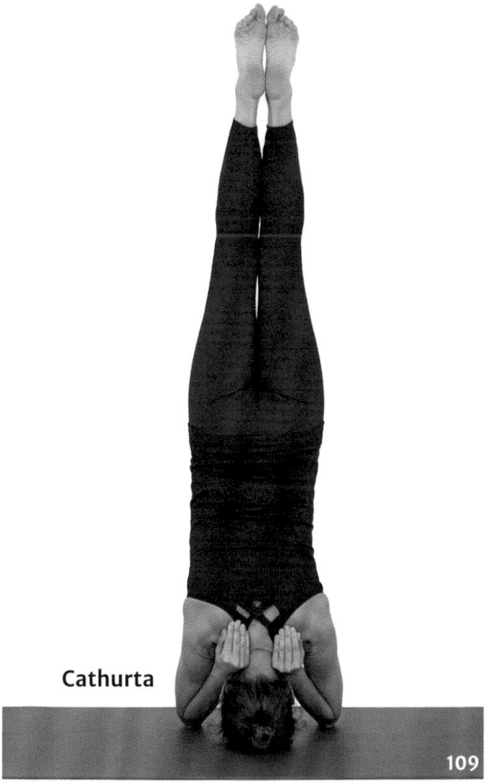
**Cathurta**

"The finishing poses, pranayama, and chanting rejuvenate the body."

Manju Jois

## Ūrdhva Dhanurāsanam ऊर्ध्व धनुरासनम्

**Samasthitiḥ** (laying down)
**Ekam** - place hands and feet in position
**Dwe** - in, come up
**Nasāgra dṛṣṭi**
**Daśa dīrgha recaka pūraka**
**Trīṇi** - ex, come down
**Catvāri** - in, come up
**Pañca** - ex, come down
**Ṣat** - in, come up
**Sapta** - ex, come down
(transition to next posture)
**Samasthitiḥ** (laying down)
**Cakrāsana**- in, roll backward
**Catvāri** - ex, caturaṅga daṇḍāsana
**Pañca** - in, ūrdhva mukha śvānāsana
**Ṣat** - ex, adho mukha śvānāsana
**Sapta** - daṇḍāsana

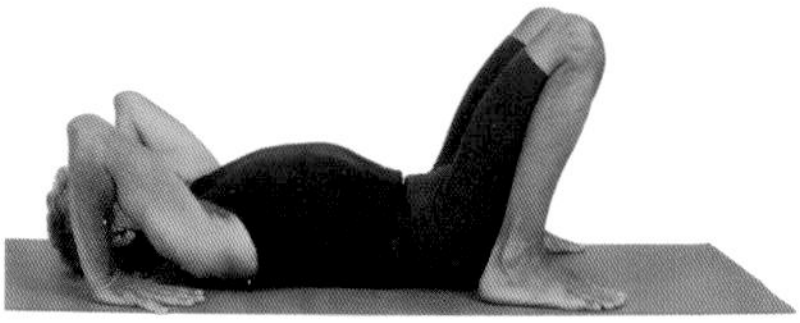

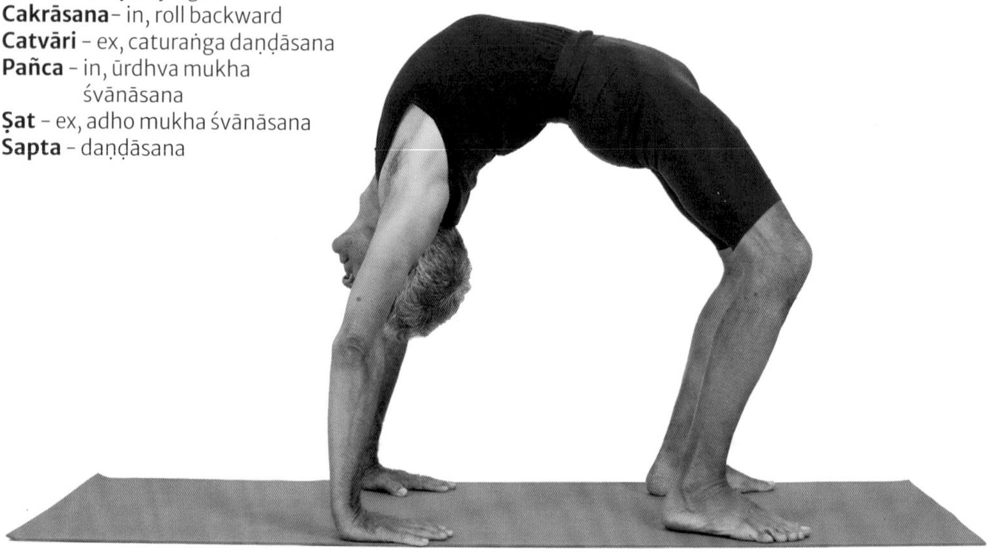

## Tṛtīya Paścimatānāsanam तृतीय पश्चिमतानासनम्

**Ekam** - bind wrist, in
**Dwe** - ex, forward bend
**Nasāgra dṛṣṭi**
**Daśa dīrgha recaka pūraka**
**Trīṇi** - in, head up
(transition to next posture)
**Catvāri** - ex, caturaṅga daṇḍāsana
**Pañca** - in, ūrdhva mukha śvānāsana
**Ṣat** - ex, adho mukha śvānāsana
**Sapta** - in, daṇḍāsana, then lay down

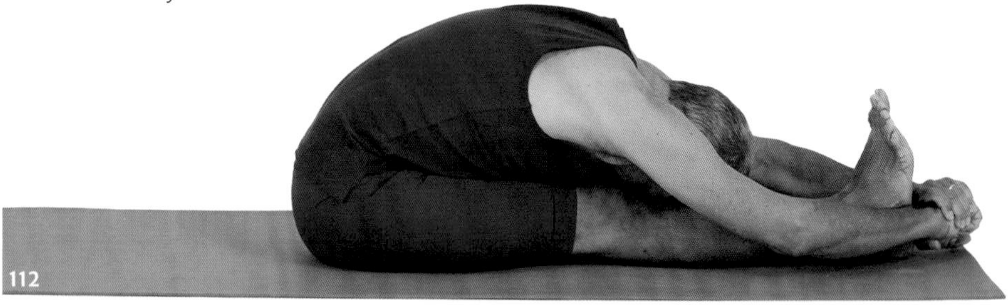

**Ekam** - in, come up
**Nasāgra dṛṣṭi**
**Daśa dīrgha recaka pūraka**

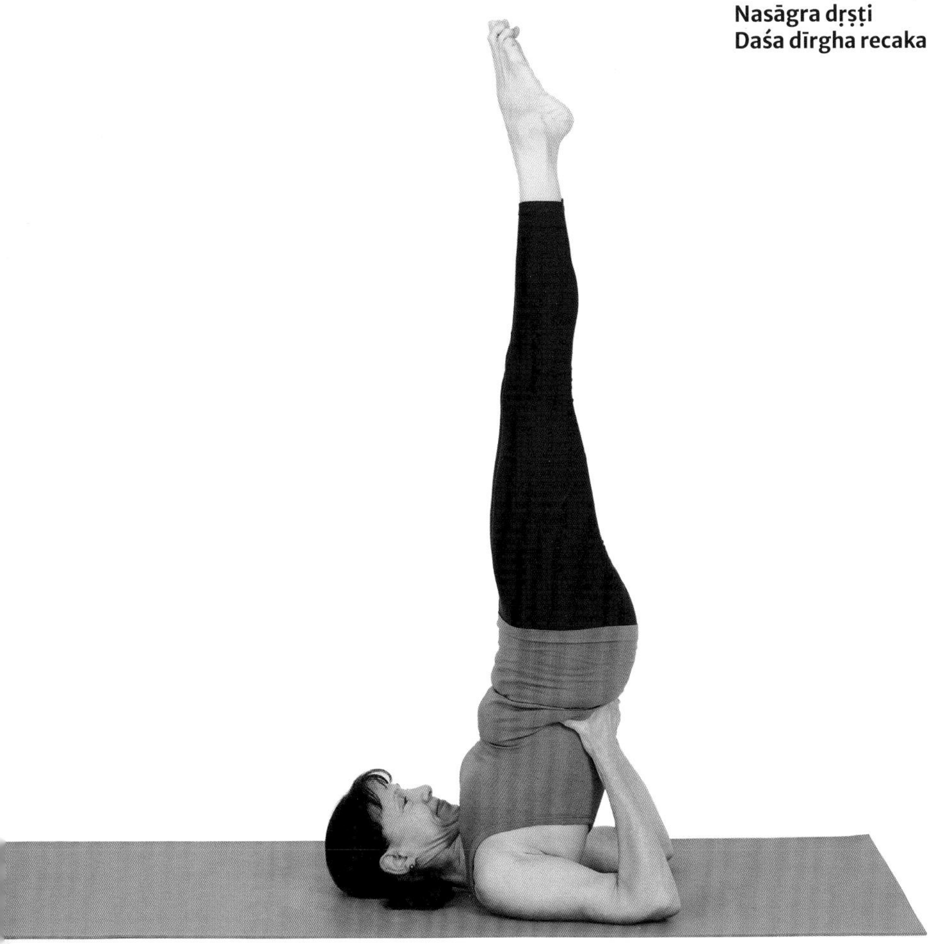

ऊर्ध्वं नाभेरधस्तालोरूर्ध्वं भानुरधः शशी । करणी
विपरीताख्या गुरुवाक्येन लभ्यते ॥ ३:७९ ॥

Ūrdhvam nābheradhastālorūrdhvam bhānuradhaḥ śaśī |
karaṇī viparītākhyā guruvākyena labhyate || 3:79 ||

Place the navel above the palate "upward the moon below the sun." This is called Viparīta Karaṇī*, it is made available by a teacher. HAṬHA YOGA PRADĪPIKA 3:79

*Refers to inverted poses. Manju recommends increasing inversions to over 5 minutes.

नाभेमूले वसेत्सूर्यस्तालुमूले च चन्द्रमाः ।
अमृतं ग्रसते सूर्यस्ततो मृत्युवशो नरः ॥ ३:२९ ॥

Nābhemūle vasetsūryastālumūle ca candramāḥ |
amṛtam grasate sūryastato mṛtyuvaśo naraḥ || 3:29 ||

In the navel root dwells *sūrya* the sun, and in the root of the palate *chandra* the moon, when *sūrya* swallows the nectar then death dwells in men. GHERAṆḌA SAMHITA 3:29

## Halāsanam — हलासनम्

**Dwe** - ex, toes together on the floor
**Nasāgra dṛṣṭi**
**Daśa dīrgha recaka**

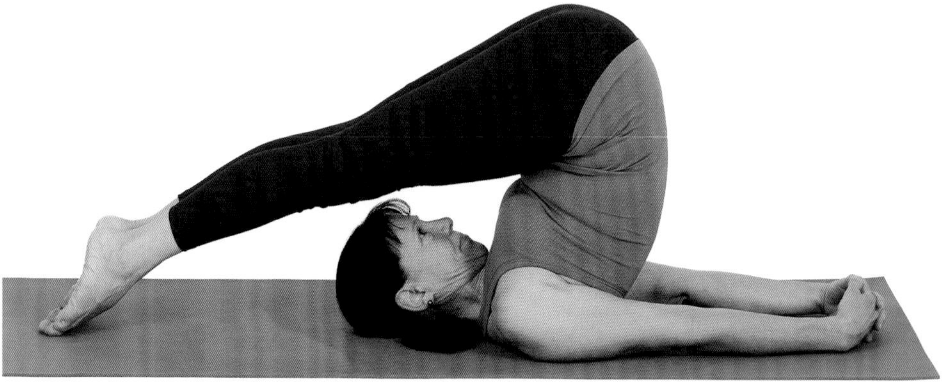

## Karṇapīḍāsanam — कर्णपीडासनम्

**Trīṇi** - ex, knees to ears
**Nasāgra dṛṣṭi**
**Daśa dīrgha recaka pūraka**

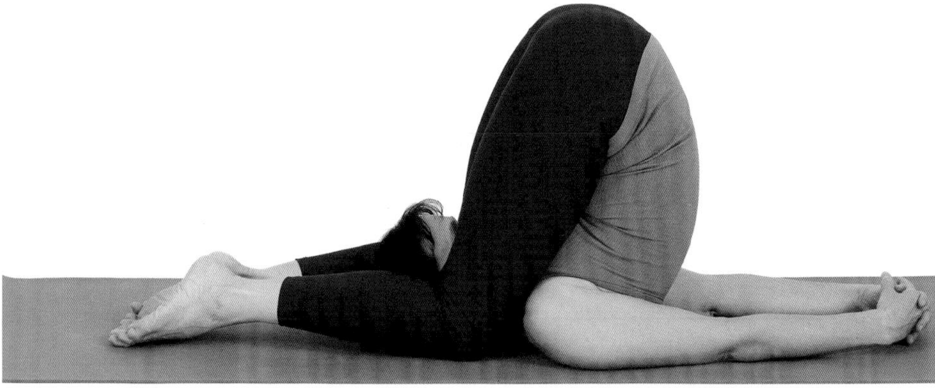

## Ūrdhva Padmāsanam ऊर्ध्व पद्मासनम्

**Catvāri** – in, sarvāṅgāsana, fold into padmāsana, hands to knees
**Nasāgra dṛṣṭi**
**Daśa dīrgha recaka pūraka**

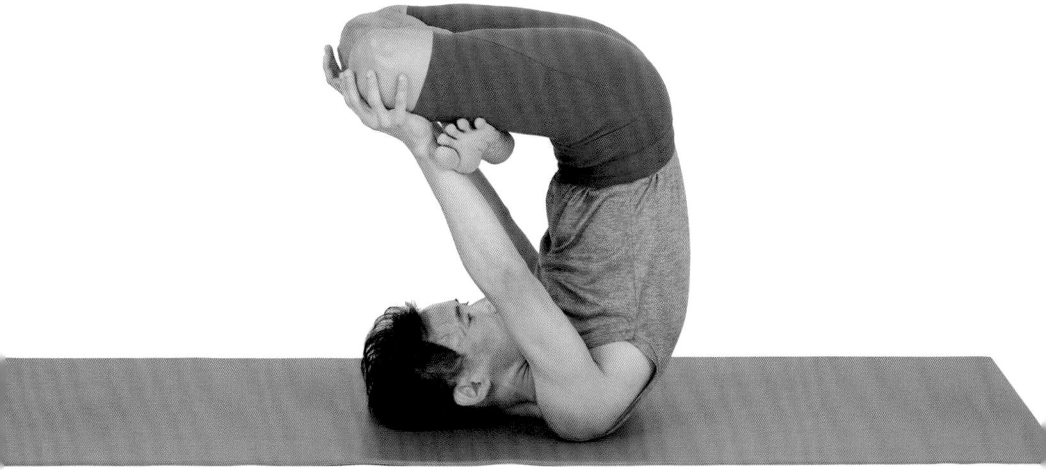

## Piṇḍāsanam पिण्डासनम्

**Pañca** – ex, knees to chest, bind the legs
**Nasāgra dṛṣṭi**
**Daśa dīrgha recaka pūraka**

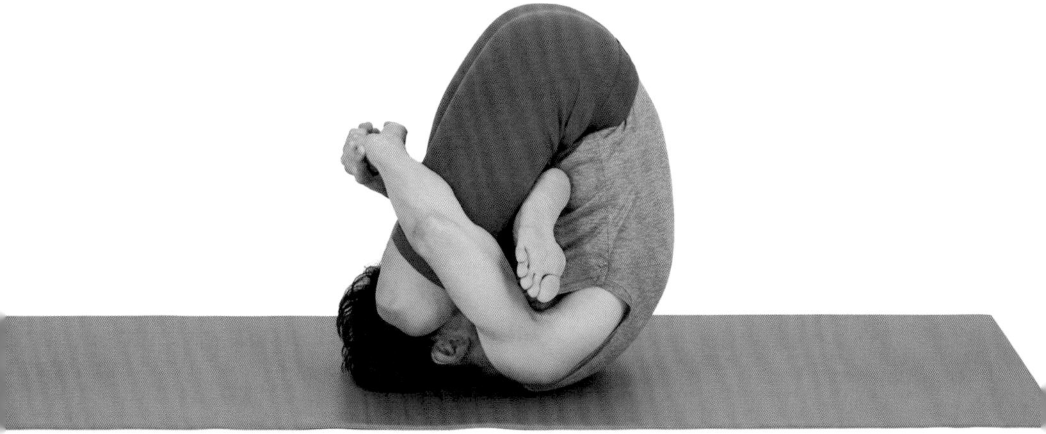

## Matsyāsanam मत्स्यासनम्

**Ṣat** - roll to the floor, place crown of head on the floor, hold the feet
**Nasāgra dṛṣṭi**
**Daśa dīrgha recaka pūraka**

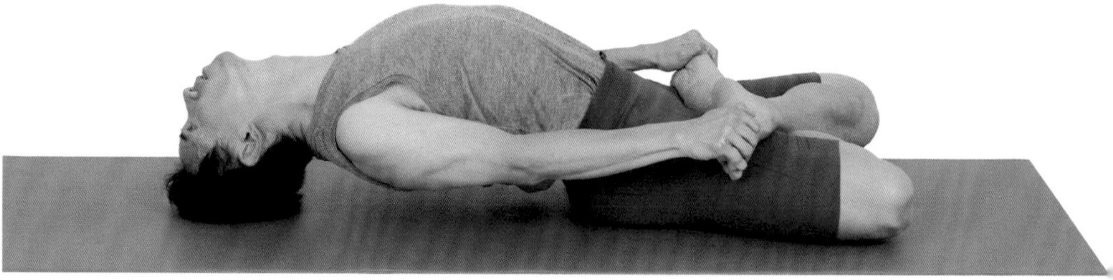

मुक्तपद्मासनं कृत्वा उत्तानशयनं चरेत् ।
कूर्पराभ्यां शिरो वेष्ट्यं मत्स्यासनं तु रोगहा ॥ २:२१ ॥

Mukta padmāsanam kṛtvā uttānaśayanam caret |
kūrparābhyām śiro veṣṭyam matsyāsanam tu rogahā || 2:21 ||

Sitting in lotus position one should lay down and enclose* the head by the elbows.
This is indeed Matsyāsana remover of diseases. GHERAṆḌA SAMHITA 2:21

*Enclose or apply pressure to the head with the elbows.

## Uttāna Pādāsanam उत्तान पादासनम्

**Sapta** - in, stretch arms and legs
**Nasāgra dṛṣṭi**
**Daśa dīrgha recaka pūraka**
**Samasthitiḥ** (lay down)
**Cakrāsana** - in, roll over the head
(or sit up and jump back)
(transition to next posture)
**Catvāri** - ex, caturaṅga daṇḍāsana
**Pañca** - in, ūrdhva mukha śvānāsana
**Ṣat** - ex, adho mukha śvānāsana
**Sapta** - baddha hasta śīrṣāsanam

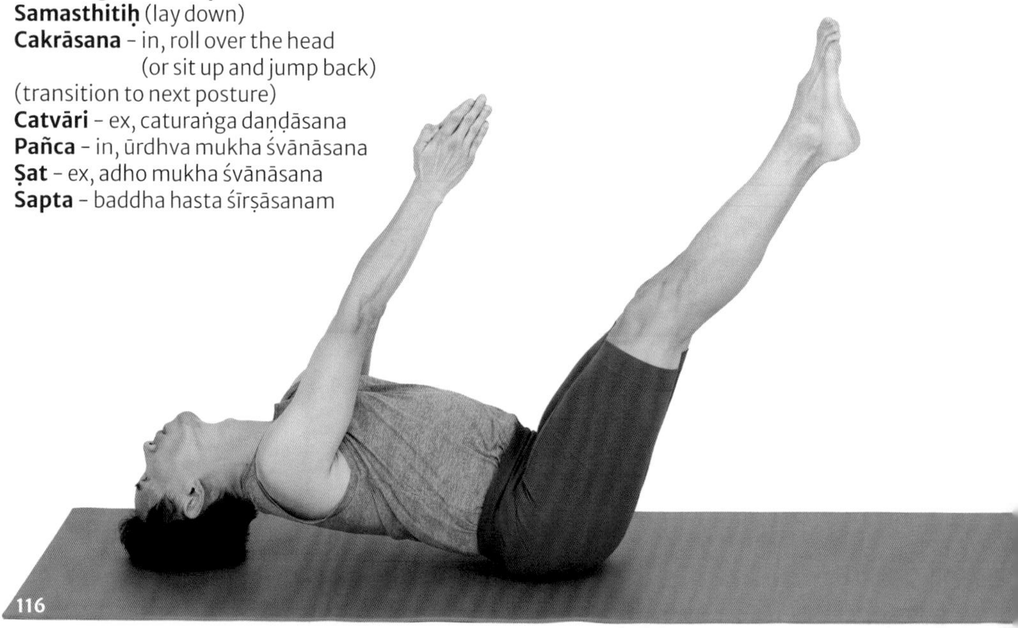

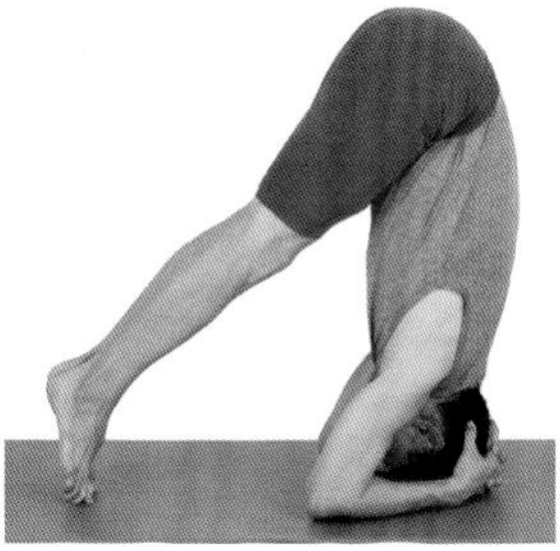

**Ekam** - knees to the floor, interlace fingers, place head
**Dwe** - in, come up
**Nasāgra dṛṣṭi**
**Daśa dīrgha recaka pūraka** *
**Trīṇi** - ex, feet to the floor, rest in balāsana

(alternate counting)
**Ekam** - knees to the floor, interlace fingers, place head
**Dwe** - in, come up
**Nasāgra dṛṣṭi**
**Daśa dīrgha recaka pūraka** *
**Trīṇi** - ex
**Ardha Candrāsanam**
**Nasāgra dṛṣṭi**
**Daśa dīrgha recaka pūraka** *
**Catvāri** - ex, Balāsanam

*When holding Śīrṣāsana do not apply pressure to top of head. Lift the head slightly off the ground, "as if a piece of paper could slide under your head." Manju Jois

3 1/2 to 5 minute holds are very therapeutic for strength and stamina.

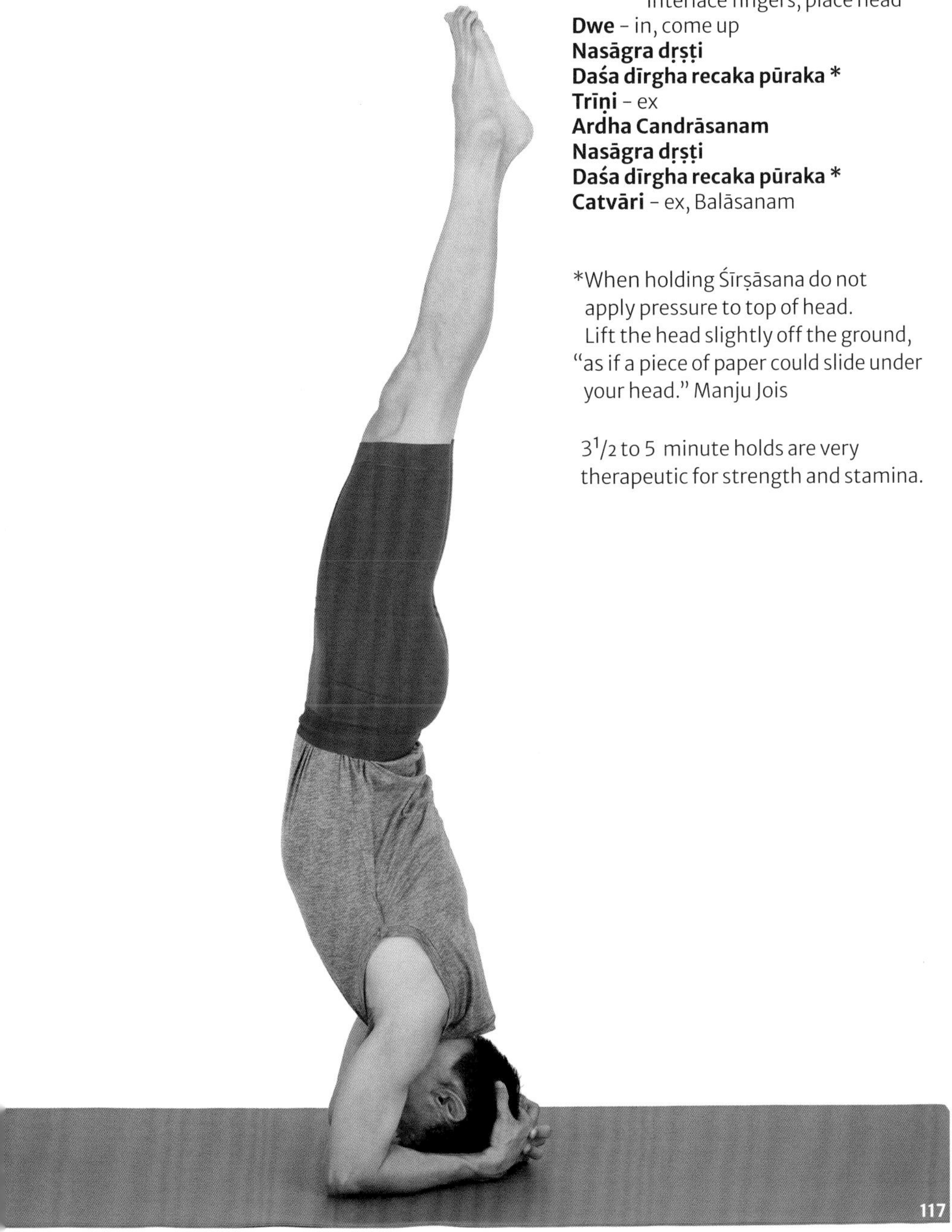

## Ardha Candrāsanam

अर्ध चन्द्रासनम्

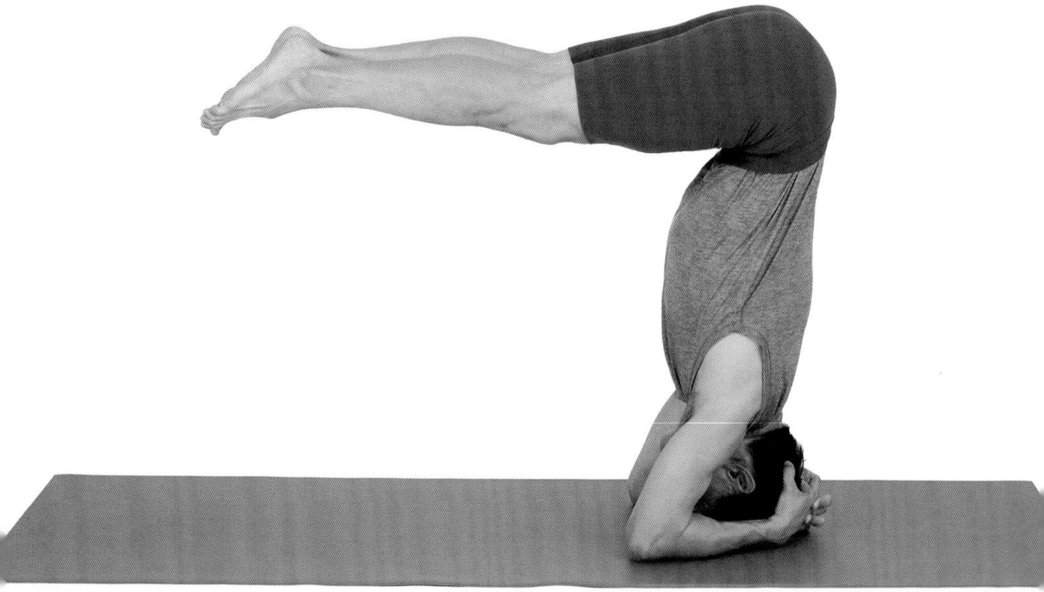

## Balāsanam

बलासनम्

Sitting on heels, forehead to floor, palms face up close to feet, or hands in front of feet, relax head and neck

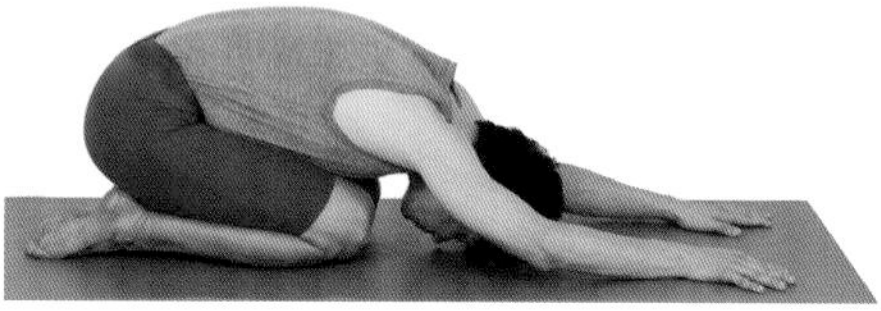

**Nasāgra dṛṣṭi**
**Daśa dīrgha recaka pūraka**
(transition to next posture)
**Catvāri** - in, place hands, ex, caturaṅga daṇḍāsana
**Pañca** - in, ūrdhva mukha śvānāsana
**Ṣat** - ex, adho mukha śvānāsana
**Sapta** - in, daṇḍāsana

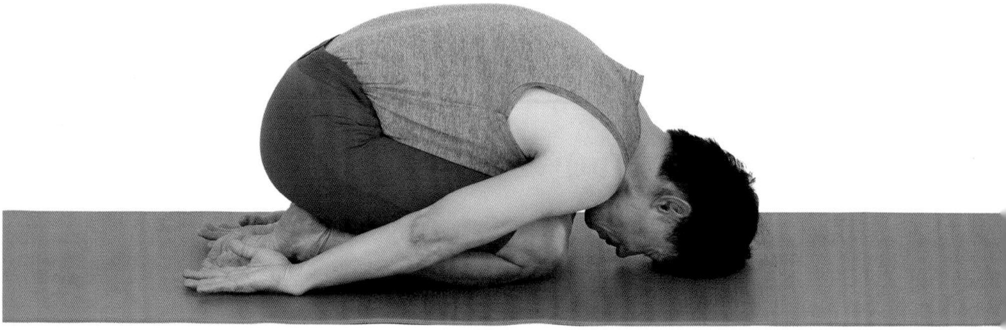

## Baddha Padmāsanam बद्ध पद्मासनम्

**Ekam** – baddha padmāsana, in

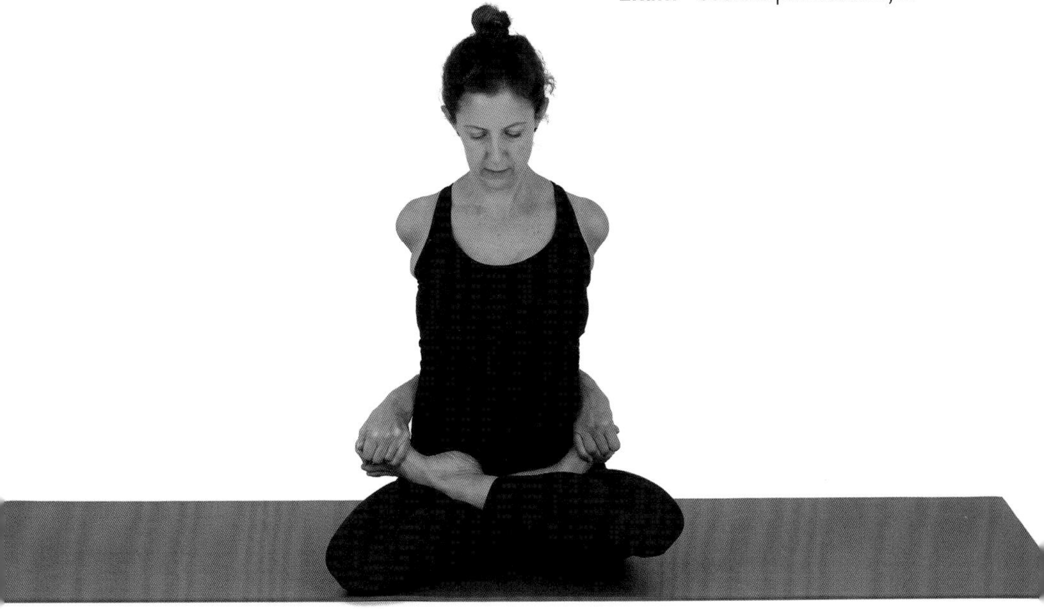

वामोरुपरि दक्षिणं च चरणं संस्थाप्य वामं तथा दक्षोरुपरि पश्चिमेन विधिना धृत्वा कराभ्यां दृढम् ।
ङ्गुष्ठौ हृदये निधाय चिबुकं नासाग्रमालोकयेदेतद्व्याधिविनाशकारि यमिनां पद्मासनं प्रोच्यते॥ १:४४ ॥

/āmorūpari dakṣinam ca caraṇam samsthāpya vāmam tathā dakṣorūpari paścimena vidhinā dhṛtvā karābhyām dṛḍham | aṅguṣṭhau hṛdaye nidhāya cibukam nāsāgramālokayedetadvyādhivināśakāri yaminām padmāsanam procyate || 1:44 ||

Bring the right foot on top of the left leg (at the hip), then the left on the right. Hold toes with hands around the back. Place the chin on the chest and focus at the tip of the nose. This Padmāsana when restrained has the power to cure disease. HAṬHA YOGA PRADĪPIKĀ 1:44

## Yoga Mudrā योग मुद्रा

**Dwe** – ex, forward bend head to floor
**Nasāgra dṛṣṭi**
**Daśa dīrgha recaka pūraka**
**Triṇi** – in, come up

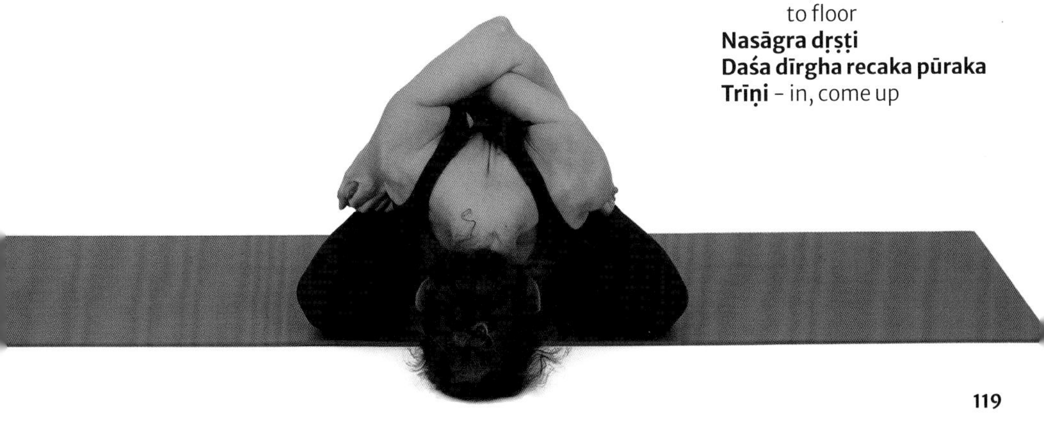

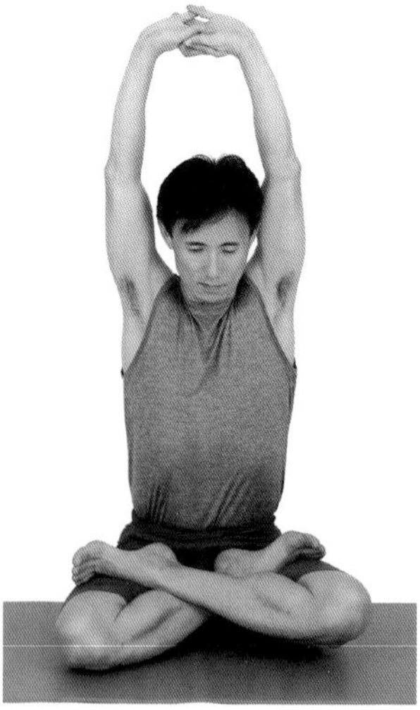

**Ekam** - in, palms above head
**Antara dṛṣṭi**
**Daśa dīrgha recaka pūraka**
**Dwe** - ex, forward bend head to floor
**Antara dṛṣṭi**
**Daśa dīrgha recaka pūraka**
**Trīṇi** - in, come up

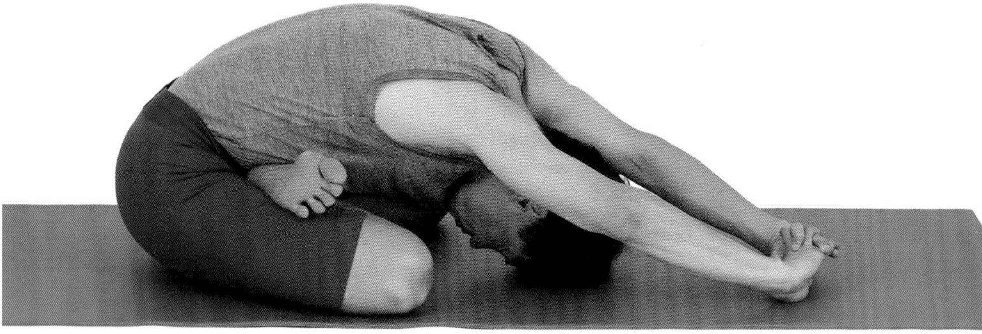

मूत्रपिण्ड यकृत् प्लीह वपाशुद्ध्यै निरन्यरम् ।
उपविश्य च सुप्ताघ पर्वतासनमभ्यसेत् ॥ २:२२ ॥

Mūtrapiṇḍa yakṛt plīha vapāśuddhai niranyaram |
upaviśya ca suptāgha parvatāsanamabhyaset || 2:22 ||

For constant cleaning of the bladder, liver, spleen, diaphragm, the organs of abdominal and thoracic cavities, one should practise Parvatāsana upright and reclined. YOGA RAHASYA 2:22

**Brūmadya dṛṣṭi**
**Daśa dīrgha recaka pūraka**

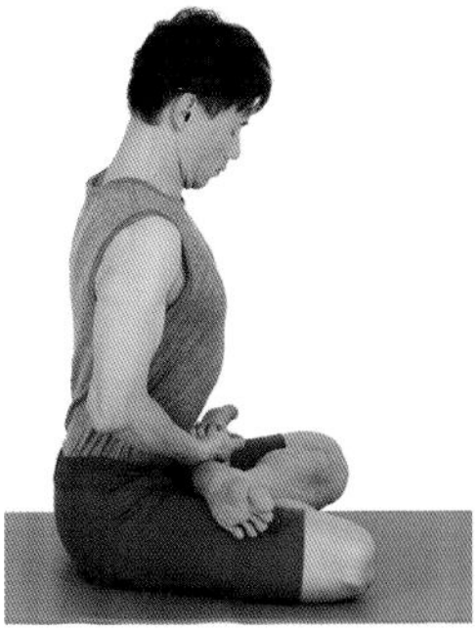

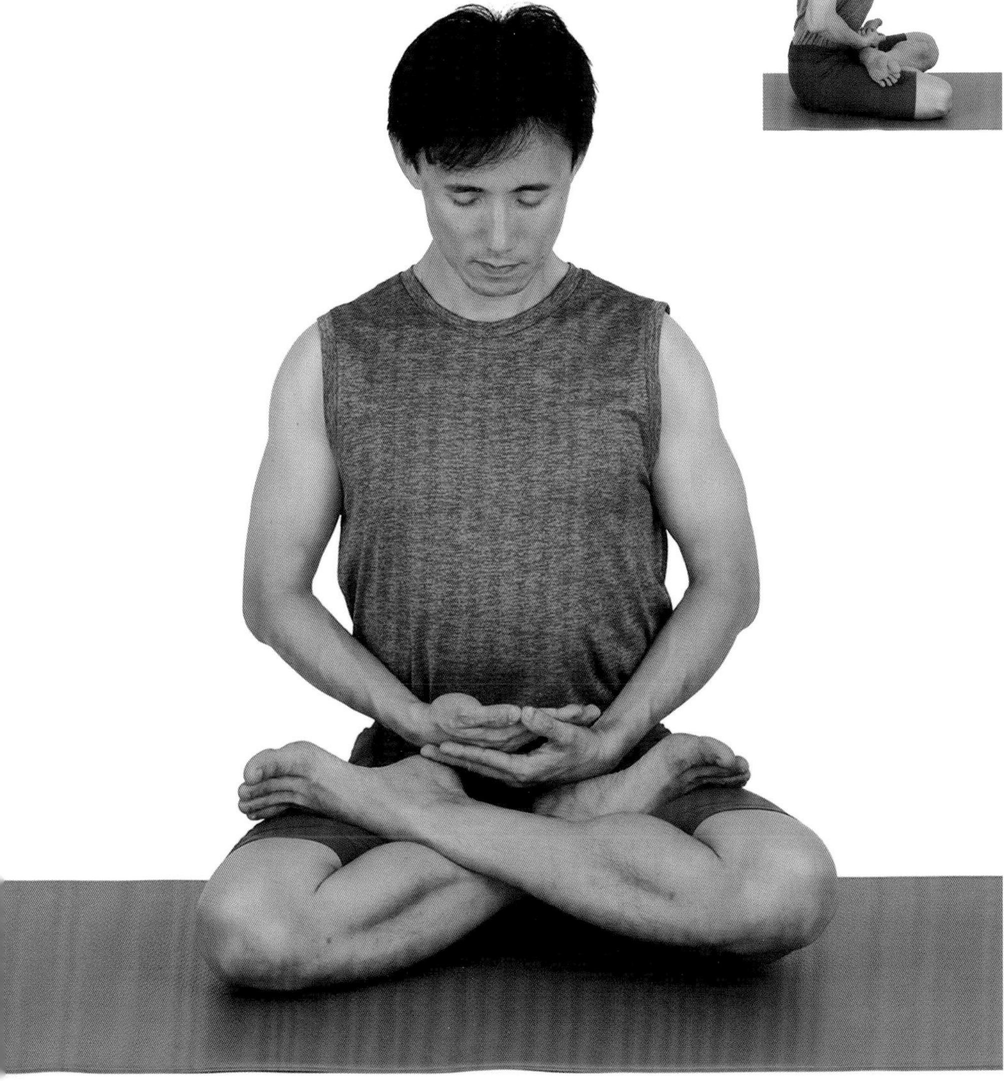

उत्तानौ चरणौ कृत्वा ऊरुसंस्थौ प्रयत्नतः ।
ऊरुमध्ये तथोत्तानौ पाणी कृत्वा ततो दृशौ ॥ १:४५ ॥

Uttānau caranau kṛtvā ūrusamsthau prayatnataḥ | ūrumadhye tathottānau pāṇī kṛtvā tato dṛṣau || 1:45 ||

Place the feet face up, secure on the thighs (in padmāsana) and the hands face up in the middle of the thighs. Gaze inward. HAṬHA YOGA PRADĪPIKĀ 1:45

**Nasāgra dṛṣṭi or Brūmadya dṛṣṭi**
(eyes closed when looking at eyebrow centre)
**Daśa dīrgha recaka pūraka**

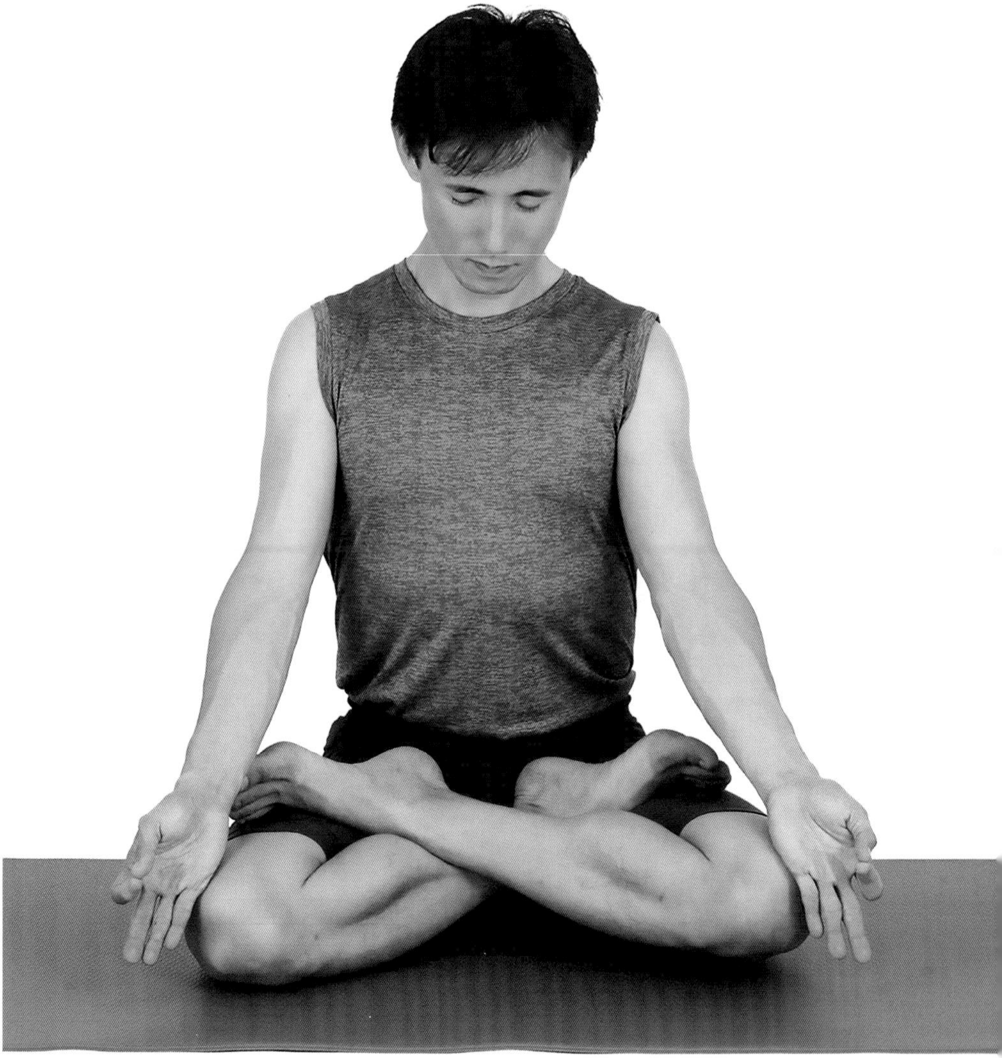

नासाग्रे विन्यसेद्राजदन्तमूले तु जिह्वया ।
उत्तम्भ्य चिबुकं वक्षस्युत्थाप्य पवनं शनैः ॥ १:४६ ॥

Nāsāgre vinyasedrājad antamūle tu jihvayā |
uttambhya cibukam vakṣasyutthāpya pavanam śanaiḥ || 1:46 ||

Place the king (attention/gaze) at the tip of the nose, the tongue on the root (upper teeth), and the chin to the upper chest. Then gradually raise the vital energy. HAṬHA YOGA PRADĪPIKĀ 1:46

## Utplutiḥ उत्प्लुतिः

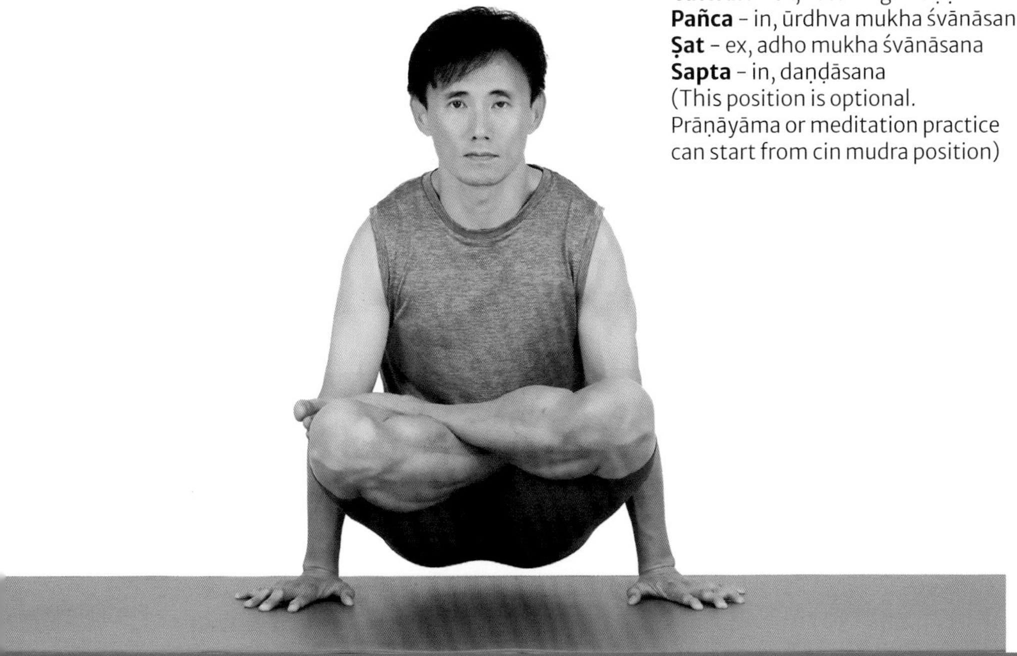

In, lift up
**Nasāgra dṛṣṭi**
**Daśa dīrgha recaka pūraka**
**Catwāri** - ex, caturaṅga daṇḍāsana
**Pañca** - in, ūrdhva mukha śvānāsana
**Ṣat** - ex, adho mukha śvānāsana
**Sapta** - in, daṇḍāsana
(This position is optional. Prāṇāyāma or meditation practice can start from cin mudra position)

## Śavāsanam शवासनम्

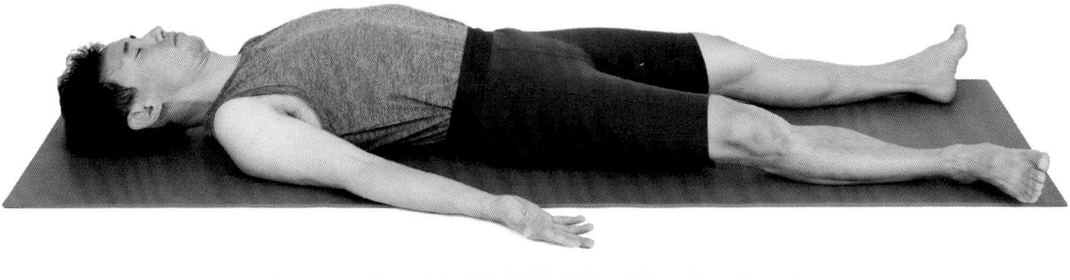

उत्तानं शववद्भूमौ शयनं तच्छवासनम् । शवासनं
श्रान्तिहरं चित्तविश्रान्तिकारकम् ॥ १:३२ ॥

Uttānam śavavad bhūmau śayanam tacchavāsanam |
śavāsanam śrāntiharam cittaviśrāntikārakam || 1:32 ||

Lay face up on the ground like a corpse in a clean position. This Śavāsana removes fatigue and calms the mind (cittam). HAṬHA YOGA PRADĪPIKĀ 1:32

"Step by step purification starts with asana, then cleansing starts with pranayama, vayu (air)."

"It is all about the process – you have to do the homework. Memorize the chanting. The sounds will saturate your brain."

Manju Jois

## आसने सुखदे योगी बद्ध्वा चैवासनं ततः ।
## दक्षनाड्या समाकृष्य बहिःस्थं पवनं शनैः ॥ २:४८ ॥

Āsane sukhade yogī baddhvā caivāsanam tataḥ |
dakṣanāḍyā samākrṣya bahiḥ stham pavanam śanaiḥ || 2:48 ||

"Sit in a comfortable yoga posture then draw air slowly through the right channel (nostril)." Haṭha Yoga Pradīpikā 2:48

## आकेशादानखाग्राच्च निरोधावधि कुम्भयेत् ।
## ततः शनैः सव्यनाड्यारेचयेत्पवनं शनैः ॥ २:४९ ॥

Ākeśādānakhāgrācca nirodhāvadhi kumbhayet |
tataḥ śanaiḥ savyanāḍyārecayetpavanam śanaiḥ || 2:49 ||

"Hold the breath after inhaling through the right nostril 'from the end of the hair to the end of the nails' then exhale through the left." Haṭha Yoga Pradīpikā 2:49

# कपालशोधनं वातदोषघ्नं कृमिदोषहृत ।
# पुनः पुनरिदं कार्यं सूर्यभेदनमुत्तमम् ॥ २:५० ॥

Kapālaśodhanam vātadoṣaghnam kṛmidoṣahṛta |
punaḥ puridam kāryam sūryabhedanamuttamam || 2:50 ||

This excellent Sūrya Bhedana cleans the skull area and fixes abdominal wind and worm problems. Haṭha Yoga Pradīpikā 2:50

**TECHNIQUE:**
First take a comfortable yogic sitting posture and start with deep sound 'Ujjayi' breathing 3–5 times. Then using the right hand, which is in Cin or Śaṅkha Mudrā, close the left nostril with the third and forth fingers and inhale slowly through the right nostril. Then with the right thumb close the right nostril and exhale slowly through the left. Holding the right thumb on the right nostril inhale through the left nostril. Close the left nostril with the third and fourth fingers and exhale through the right nostril. Repeat 3–5 times.

**RETENTION:**
Breathe in deeply through the right nostril; at the pinnacle of the inhale bring the hands to the knees, straighten the spine, and place the chin on the collarbones. Hold the breath (kumbhaka) for 15–20 seconds. Then close the right nostril with the right thumb and exhale slowly through left nostril. Keep the right nostril closed with the thumb and inhale through the left nostril. At the pinnacle of the inhale bring the hands to the knees, straighten the spine, and place the chin on the collarbones. Hold the breath (kumbhaka) for 15–20 seconds. Close the left nostril with the third and fourth fingers and exhale through the right nostril. Repeat this cycle 3–5 times.

**CAUTION:**
Prāṇāyāma exercises should be approached with care and consistency. Beginners should not hold the kumbhakas longer than 15 counts when first starting breath retention. Over many months or years, one can build up to 35 counts.

Additionally, Sūrya Bhedana Prāṇāyāma can be performed using only the right nostril. Manju generally does not teach this variation. If performed it is best done with minimal holding of the kumbhaka on extremely cold days to warm the body.

**BENEFITS:**
This prāṇāyāma is particularly helpful in clearing out the frontal sinus cavities. Sūrya Bhedana translates as "sun piercing." It also alleviates congestion in the nasal/sinus cavities.

Performed slowly without forcing the kumbhaka (retention) it is very soothing for the nervous system.

Manju says this Prāṇāyāma brings seratonin to the brain.

Increasing the kumbhaka will bring up the heat in the body and help clarify physical and mental blockages.

According to Swātmārāma in Haṭha Yoga Pradīpikā, it also helps eradicate abdominal worms.

सीत्कां कुर्यात्तथा वक्त्रे घ्राणेनैव विजृंभिकाम् ।
एवमभ्यासयोगेन कामदेवो द्वितीयकः ॥ २:५४ ॥

Sītkām kuryāttathā vaktre ghrāṇenaiva vijṛmbhikām |
evamabhyāsayogena kāmadevo dwitīyakaḥ || 2:50 ||

"Sītkām (Sitkari prāṇāyāma) is performed thus. Breathe into the mouth, which is opened wide (with teeth together) as if one was yawning. Through this yoga practice they become a second Kāmadeva." Haṭha Yoga Pradīpika 2:50

**TECHNIQUE:**
Begin in a comfortable seated yoga position and take five deep 'Ujjāyī' breaths. Then exhale through the mouth while leaning forward towards the floor. Next inhale over the teeth through a wide open mouth while straightening the spine. At the top of the inhale, apply kumbhaka and hold for a few seconds, then exhale through the nostrils while leaning forward towards the floor. Repeat 3–5 times.

Finish as you started with 3–5 five deep breaths.

**BENEFITS:**
Manju highlights this technique to maintain good gum hygiene and to calm and/or cool the body.

Swātmārāma says through this prāṇāyāma one can become a second Kamadeva, who is the "god of love." This teaching can simply be that the body of someone who is a prāṇāyāma (and āsana) adept becomes slim, beautiful and primed for success (above śloka).

...कास्यस्य कृशता कान्ति तदा जायेत् निश्चितम्

...kāsyasya kṛśatā kāntitadā jāyet niścitam

...the body becomes slim, beautiful and certain of success. Haṭha Yoga Pradīpika 2:29

The inhale through the teeth and mouth can also be felt in the face and neck. This relaxes the facial musculature and stimulates the neck and cranial nerves to refresh the whole head. Additionally, this stimulates the meridian system connected to the eyes, ears, nose and tongue.

## जिह्वया वायुमाकृष्य पूर्ववत् कुंभसाधनम् । शनकैर्घ्राणरन्ध्राभ्यां रेचयेत् पवनं सुधीः ॥ २:५८ ॥

Jihvyā vāyumākṛṣya pārvavat kumbhasādhanam |
śanakairghrāṇarandhrābhyām recayet pavanam sudhīḥ || 2.58 ||

"Plough (inhale) the air through the tongue and perform kumbhaka. The wise will then slowly exhale through both nostrils." Haṭha Yoga Pradīpika 2:58

## गुल्मप्लीहादिकान् रोगाञ्ज्वरं पित्तं क्षुधां तृषाम् । विषाणि शीतली नाम कुंभिकेयं निहन्ति हि ॥ २:५९ ॥

Gulmaplihādikān rogāñjvram pittam kṣudhām tṛṣām |
viṣāṇi śītalī nāma kumbhikeyam nihanti hi || 2:59 ||

"Indeed Śitalī has curative effects (destroying) distension and spasms of the abdomen, enlargement of the spleen, fever, issues with bile, hunger, thirst, poisons and eye diseases." Haṭha Yoga Pradīpika 2:59

## सर्वदा साधयेद्योगी शीतलीकुंभकं शुभम् । अजीर्णं कफपित्तं च नैव तस्य प्रजायते ॥ ५:७४ ॥

Sarvadā sādhayedyogī śītalīkumbhakam śubham |
ajīrṇam kaphapittam ca naiva tasya prajāyate || 5:74 ||

"Once the yogi is consistently practicing Śitalī kumbhaka they are the beneficiaries of strong digestion and a lack of Pitta and Kapha disorders." Gheraṇḍa Samhita 5:74

**TECHNIQUE:**
Sit in a comfortable seated position. Start with 5 deep breaths, then curl the tongue so a channel is formed along the whole length. Exhale through the curled tongue while leaning forward towards the floor and squeeze all the air out of the lungs. Then inhale through the curled tongue towards the ceiling. Hold the breath for a few seconds, then exhale through the nostrils. Repeat 3-5 times. Finish with 5 deep breaths through the nostrils.

**Caution:** Kumbhaka in Śitalī prāṇāyāma should only be held momentarily. The emphasis should be on a long inhale and exhale.

**BENEFITS:**
Manju says that the main benefit of this prāṇāyāma is the cooling of the body. This is a safe yogic practice when one has a light fever or excessive heat. One should contact one's health care provider if these symptoms persist or are debilitating.

Swātmārāma says that this prāṇāyāma has a number of curative benefits. In Ayurvedic medicine the shape, color, and health of the tongue is a direct reflection of the health and metabolic state of the torso and head. "Ploughing" the tongue with air will "feed back" into the body's metabolic state and provide curative effects as listed in the ślokas listed above.

## सम्यक्पद्मासनं बद्ध्वा समग्रीवोदरं सुधीः ।
## मुखं संयम्य यत्नेन प्राणं घ्राणेन रेचयेत् ॥ २:६० ॥

Samyakpadmāsanam baddhvā samagrīvodaram sudhīḥ |
mukham samyamya yatnena prāṇam ghrāṇena recayet || 2:60 ||

"The wise should sit in padmāsana, align the stomach and neck while closing the mouth. Then with effort exhale through the nose." Haṭha Yoga Pradīpikā 2:60

## यथा लगति हृत्कण्ठे कपालावधि सस्वनम् ।
## वेगेन पूरयेच्चापि हृत्पद्मावधि मारुतम् ॥ २:६१ ॥

Yathā lagati hṛtkanṭhe kapālāvadhi sasvanam |
vegena pūrayeccāpi hṛtpadmāvadhi mārutam || 2:61 ||

"Then breathe in forcefully (through both nostrils) with sound into the heart, throat and skull." Hatha Yoga Pradipika 2:61

## पुनर्विरेचयेत्तद्वत् पूरयेच्च पुनः पुनः ।
## यथैव लोहकारेण भस्त्रा वेगेन चाल्यते ॥ २:६२ ॥

Punarvirecayettadvat pūrayecca punaḥ punaḥ |
Yathaiva lohakāreṇa bhastrā vegena cālyate || 2:62 ||

"It is done again and again pumping the breath in and out like the blacksmith and his bellows." Haṭha Yoga Pradīpika 2:62

**TECHNIQUE:**
Sit in a comfortable seated position or Padmāsana.
Start with 5 deep breaths.
With effort exhale fully until the stomach muscles are tightened.
Hold the toes, then inhale and exhale forcefully, approximately 10 times.
Then inhale fully, straighten the spine, and perform kumbhaka.
Hold for 15-20 seconds.
Repeat steps 1-3.

Finish with 5 deep Ujjāyī breaths.

**CAUTION:**
Bhastrikā is a strong prāṇāyāma. It should be learned carefully, and beginners should not use too much force when first practicing the prāṇāyāma. The inhales and exhales need to be approximately the same length. One should also have an empty stomach when performing this prāṇāyāma.

**BENEFITS:**
The belly movement acts to stimulate the digestion and Jaṭhara Agni, the digestive fire.

The rush of air benefits the sinus cavities and helps clear mucus from nasal passages.

Bhastrikā invigorates and can be performed in the morning to stimulate the metabolism.

जलेन श्रमजातेन गात्रमर्दनमाचरेत् ।
दृधता लघुता चैव तेन गात्रस्य जायते ॥ २:१३ ॥

Jalena śramajātena gātramardanamācaret |
dṛdhatā laghutā caiva tena gātrasya jāyate || 2:13 ||

The massage of yoga produced sweat into the limbs, brings forth firmness, lightness and victory." Haṭha Yoga Pradīpikā 2:13.

Practitioners of prāṇāyāma and/or intense āsanas are likely to sweat a great deal in the beginning. This is a detoxification process and minimizes over time. The sweat of a healthy Haṭha yogi contains much that is healthy for the body. Rubbing the sweat back into the body reincorporates these into the body.

"Chanting is very powerful. That is why we need to chant every day. The slow vibration purifies you. If you hear nice chanting, your mind reacts to it positively. The vibration starts in your head and that is what clears up the cloud in your mind. Everyone has a cloud sitting there (in their head) so we must help make it disappear. The sun is behind the cloud. The chanting brings the sun. It is called Atman in Sanskrit—it means your soul and jnana means knowledge—you will see the whole knowledge come out of you. And that is what we are trying to discover. It comes with daily action."

Manju Jois

ओं सह नाववतु । सह नौ भनक्तु ।
सह वीर्यम् करवावहै । तेजस्विनावधीतमस्तु मा विद्विषावहै ॥
ओं शान्तिः शान्तिः शान्तिः ॥

om saha nāvavatu | saha nau bhunaktu |
saha vīryam karavāvahai |
tejasvināvadhītamastu mā vidviṣāvahai ||
om śāntiḥ śāntiḥ śāntiḥ ||

May Brahman protect us both together, may he nourish us both together.
May we both work together with great energy.
May our study be vigorous and effective. May we never hate each other.
May peace – physical, mental and spiritual be on us forever.

ओं शं नो मित्रः शं वरुणः। शं नो भवत्वर्यमा। शं न इन्द्रो बृहस्पतिः । शं नो विष्णुरुरुक्रमः। नमो ब्रह्मणे नमस्ते वायो । त्वमेव प्रत्यक्षं ब्रह्मासि । त्वामेव प्रत्यक्षं ब्रह्मवदिष्यामि । ऋतं वदिष्यामि । सत्यं वदिष्यामि । तन्मामवतु । तद्वक्तारमवतु । अवतु माम् । अवतु वक्तारम् ॥ ओं शान्तिः शान्तिः शान्तिः ॥

Om śan no mitraḥ śam varuṇaḥ । śan no bhavatvaryamā । śan na indro bṛhaspatiḥ । śan no viṣṇururukramaḥ । namo brahmaṇe । namaste vāyo । tvameva pratyakṣam brahmāsi । tvāmeva pratyakṣam brahma vadiṣyāmi । ṛtam vadiṣyāmi । satyam vadiṣyāmi । tanmāmavatu । tadvaktāramavatu । avatu mām । avatu vaktāram ॥ Om śāntiḥ śāntiḥ śāntiḥ ॥

May Mitra (the sun who controls the Prana) grant us peace; May Varuna (the Lord of the night and controller of the Apana) grant peace to us; May Aryaman (the Principle of chivalry) be propitious to us; May Indra (the cosmic mind) and Brihaspati (the principle of wisdom) grant us peace; May Vishnu of great strides (the Supreme omnipresent Godhead) be propitious to us; Salutations to you, Brahman (the absolute reality), and salutations to Vayu (the life-force of the universe). You alone are the perceptible Brahman. You alone I shall proclaim to be the perceptible Godhead. I shall speak of the right, I shall speak of the truth. May that (teaching) protect me and also the preceptor. Let that protect us both, the taught and the teacher. Om, let there be peace all pervading.

ओं भद्रं कर्णेभिः शृणुयाम देवाः । भद्रं पश्येमाक्षभिर्यजत्राः ।
स्थिरैरङ्गैस्तुष्टुवागंसस्तनूभिः । व्यशेम देवहितं यदायुः ।
स्वस्ति न इन्द्रो वृद्धश्रवाः । स्वस्ति नः पूषाविश्ववेदाः ।
स्वस्ति नो तार्क्ष्यो अरिष्टनेमिः । स्वस्ति नो बृहस्पतिर्दधातु ॥
ओं शान्तिः शान्तिः शान्तिः ॥

Om bhadram karṇebhiḥ śṛṇuyāma devāḥ । bhadram paśyemākṣbhiryajatrāḥ । sthirairaṅgaistuṣṭuvāgmsastanūbhiḥ । vyaśema devahitaṁ yadāyuḥ । swasti na indro vṛddhaśravāḥ । swasti naḥ pūṣā viśvavedāḥ । swasti no tārkṣyo ariṣṭanemiḥ । swasti no bṛhaspatirdadhātu ॥ Om śāntiḥ śāntiḥ śāntiḥ ॥

O Gods, while engaged in sacrifices, may we hear with our ears what is auspicious, may we see with our eyes what is auspicious. While praising, may we be of strong and steady limb, enjoy life given by the gods, may Indra of ancient fame be blissful to us; May Garuda, the destroyer of evil be blissful to us, may Brhaspati be blissful to us. Om peace peace peace.

ओं नमो ब्रह्मणे नमो अस्त्वग्नये नमः पृथिव्यै नम ओषधिभ्यः ।
नमो वाचे नमो वाचस्पतये नमो विष्णवे बृहते करोमि ॥
ओं शान्तिः शान्तिः शान्तिः ॥

Om namo brahmaṇe namo astvagnaye namaḥ pṛthivyai nama oṣadhībhyaḥ । namo vāce namo vācaspataye namo viṣṇave bṛhate karomi ॥ Om śāntiḥ śāntiḥ śāntiḥ ॥

Salutations to Brahma, salutations to Agni, salutations to the earth, salutations to the medicinal plants, salutations to Speech, salutations to the master of speech, salutations to Vishnu, to the great mystic one, I do salute. Om peace peace peace.

ओं तच्छं योरावृणीमहे । गातुं यज्ञाय । गातुं यज्ञपतये ।
दैवी स्वस्तिरस्तु नः। स्वस्तिर्मानुषेभ्यः । ऊर्ध्वं जिगातु भेषजम् ।
शं नो अस्तु द्विपदे । शं चतुष्पदे ॥ ओं शान्तिः शान्तिः शान्तिः ॥

Om tacchaṁ yorāvṛnīmahe । gātum yajñāya । gātum yajñapataye । daivī swastirastu naḥ । swastirmānuṣebhyaḥ । ūrdhvam jigātu bheṣajam । śan no astu dvipade । śan catuṣpade ॥ Om śāntiḥ śāntiḥ śāntiḥ ॥

We worship the Supreme Person for the welfare of all. May all miseries and shortcomings leave us forever so that we may always chant in the sacrifices and for the Lord of Sacrifices. May the medicinal herbs grow in potency so that diseases can be cured effectively. May the devas grant us peace. May all human beings be happy, may all the birds and the beasts also be happy. Om peace, peace, peace.

ओं यश्छन्दसामृषभो विश्वरूपः । छन्दोभ्योऽध्यमृताथ्सम्बभूव । स मेन्द्रो मेधया स्पृणोतु । अमृतस्य देवधारणो भूयासम् । शरीरं मे विचर्षणम् । जिह्वा मे मधुमत्तमा ।कर्णाभ्यां भूरिविश्रुवम् । ब्रह्मणः कोशोऽसि मेधया पिहितः । श्रुतं मे गोपाय ॥ ओं शान्तिः शान्तिः शान्तिः ॥

Om yaśchandasāmṛṣabho vishvarūpaḥ । chandobhyo'dhyamṛtāthsambabhūva । sa mendro medhayā spṛnotu । amṛtasya devadhārano bhūyāsam । śarīram me vicarṣaṇam । jihvā me madhumattamā । karṇābhyām bhūriviśruvam । brahmanaḥ kosho'si medhayā pihitaḥ । śrutam me gopāya ॥ Om śāntiḥ śāntiḥ śāntiḥ ॥

May He who is the bull of the Vedic hymns, who assumes all forms, who has sprung from the immortal hymns of the Vedas – may the Supreme Lord strengthen me with wisdom. May I, O God, become an upholder of the immortal revelation. May I be able and active in body, may my speech be sweet and agreeable to the highest degree, may I hear abundant (teachings) with my ears. You, O AUM, are the veil of Brahman, which is concealed within me by my intellect. May whatever I have learned be preserved. Om peace peace peace.

ओं पूर्णमदः पूर्णमिदं पूर्णात् पूर्णमुदच्यते । पूर्णस्य पूर्णमादाय । पूर्णमेवावशिष्यते ॥ ओं शान्तिः शान्तिः शान्तिः ॥

Om pūrṇamadaḥ pūrṇamidam pūrṇat pūrṇamudacyate । pūrṇasya pūrṇamādāya pūrṇamevāvaśiṣyate ॥ Om śāntiḥ śāntiḥ śāntiḥ ॥

That (Supreme Being) is perfect; this (Jiva) is perfect. From the perfect, the perfect arises. Taking the perfect from the perfect, the perfect alone remains. Om peace peace peace. Translation: Rami Śivan

ओं असतो मा सद्गमय । तमसो मा ज्योतिर्गमय । मृत्योर्माऽमृतं गमय ॥ ओं शान्तिः शान्तिः शान्तिः ॥

Om asato mā sadgamaya । tamaso mā jyotirgamaya । mrtyormā'mṛtam gamaya ॥ Om śāntiḥ śāntiḥ śāntiḥ ॥

From untruth, lead us to truth. From ignorance, lead us to wisdom. From death, lead us to immortality. Om peace peace peace. Translation: Rami Śivan

ओं प्रणमस्य परब्रह्म ऋषिः परमात्मा देवता देवी गायत्री छन्दः प्राणायामे विनियोगः ॥

ओं भूः । ओं भुवः । ओं सुवः । ओं महः । ओं जनः । ओं तपः । ओं सत्यं । ओं तथ्सवितुर्वरेण्यं भर्गो देवस्य धीमहि । धियो यो नः प्रचोदयात् । ओं आपो ज्योतीरसोऽमृतं ब्रह्म भूर् भुवः सुवरोम् ॥ ओं शान्तिः शान्तिः शान्तिः ॥

Om praṇamasya* parabrahma ṛṣiḥ paramātmā devatā devī gāyatrī chandaḥ prāṇāyāme viniyogaḥ ॥

Om bhūḥ । Om bhuvaḥ । Om suvaḥ । Om mahaḥ । Om janaḥ । Om tapaḥ । Om satyam । Om tathsaviturvareṇyam bhargo devasya dhīmahi । dhiyo yo naḥ pracodayāt । Om āpo jyotī raso'mṛitam brahma bhūr bhuvaḥ suvarom ॥ Om śāntiḥ śāntiḥ śāntiḥ ॥

Om, The material world,
Om, The realm of mind,
Om, The realm of light,
Om, The realm of vastness,
Om, The realm of creative delight,
Om, The realm of unobstructed will,
Om, The realm of the highest truth,

Om, May we meditate upon that Adorable Light of the Divine Creator, and may He enlighten our intellect.

Om, He is in the water, light, flavor, nectar of immortality and also pervades the three realms-physical, mental and spiritual.
He who is denoted by Praṇava is all these.

* alternative: praṇavasya

ओं स्वस्ति प्रजाभ्याम् परिपालयन्ताम् ।
न्यायेन मार्गेण महीं महीशाः।
गो ब्राह्मणेभ्याश्च शुभमस्तु नित्यं ।
लोखाः समस्ताः सुखिनो भबन्तु ॥

Om swasti prajābhyām* paripālayantām ।
nyāyena mārgena mahīm mahīśāḥ ।
go brāhmanebhyāśca* śubhamastu nityam ।
lokhāḥ samastāḥ sukhino bhavantu ॥

May it be well with the protector of the progeny on earth, And let them lead with intelligence for a peaceful earth, May it be well with the connection between us and permanence. May it be well with all beings everywhere.

सर्वे जन सुखिनो भवन्तु । समस्त संमङ्गलानिसन्तु ।
लोक कल्यान संवृत्तिरस्तु । विश्वशान्तिरस्तु ॥
ओं शान्तिः शान्तिः शान्तिः ॥

Sarve jana sukhino bhavantu । samasta sanmaṅgalānisantu । loka kalyāṇa samvṛttirastu viśvaśāntirastu ॥ Om śāntiḥ śāntiḥ śāntiḥ ॥

In all births let there be happiness, may auspiciousness be everywhere, let there be well-being for all, let there be peace everywhere. Om peace peace peace.

* alternate: prajābhyāḥ, brāhmanebhyāḥ

## Ganesh

ओं गणानां त्वा गणपतिगं् हवामहे कविं कवीनामुपमश्रवस्तमम् ।
ज्येष्ठराजं ब्रह्मणां ब्रह्मनस्पत आ नः शृण्वन्नूतिभिस्सीद सादनम् ॥
ओं श्री महा गणपतये नमः

Om gaṇānān tvā gaṇapatigm havāmahe kāvin kavīnām upamaśravastamam । jyeṣṭharājam brahmaṇām brahmaṇaspata ā naḥ śṛṇvannūtibhissīda sādanam ॥ Om śrī mahā gaṇapataye namaḥ ॥

O Lord of Hosts we invoke you, Sage of sages, most famous. The highest King of the enlightened, O Lord of prayer, hearken to us, respond and be present here in your appointed place. Translation Rami Śivan

ओं शुक्लाम्बरधरं विष्णुं शशिवर्णं चतुर्भुजं । प्रसन्नवदनं ध्यायेत् सर्व विघ्नोपशान्तये ॥

Om śuklāmbaradharam viṣṇum śaśivarṇam caturbhujam ।
prasannavadanam dhyāyet sarva vighnopaśāntaye ॥

One should meditate for the removal of all obstacles upon Viṣṇu who is clad in white garments, who has a lustre like the moon, who has four arms and a beneficent face. Translation Rami Śivan

## Shiva

ओं त्र्यंबकं यजामहे सुगन्धिं पुष्टिवर्धनम् ।
ऊर्वारुकमिवबंधान्मृत्योर्मुक्षीय माऽमृतात् ॥

Om tryambakam yajāmahe sugamdhim puṣṭivardhanam । ūrvārukamiva bandhānmṛtyor mukṣīya mā'mṛtāt ॥

We salute and venerate the three-eyed One, who is perfumed, who increases the wellbeing of his devotees. May He liberate us from death [and rebirth], like the cucumber from its stalk, and establish us firmly on the path to Liberation. Translation: Rami Śivan

## Three Gurus

ओं गुरुर्ब्रह्मा गुरुर्विष्णुः गुरुर्देवो महेश्वरः । गुरु साक्षात् परब्रह्म तस्मै श्रीगुरुवे नमः ॥

Om gururbrahmā gururviṣnuḥ gururdevo maheśvaraḥ ।
guru sākṣāt parabrahma tasmai śrī guruve namaḥ ॥

Salutations to that glorious guru who is the manifestation of the creating, preserving and transforming energies of the cosmos. The guru is himself that Supreme Being. Translation: Rami Śivan

**Krishna**

जयतु जयतु देवो देवकीनन्दनोऽयं । जयतु जयतु कृष्णो वृष्णिवम्शप्रदीपः । जयतु जयतु मेघश्यामलः कोमलाङ्गः । जयतु जयतु कृष्णो भारनाशो मुकुन्दः ॥ ३ ॥

Jayatu jayatu devo devakīnandano'yam । jayatu jayatu kṛṣṇo vṛṣṇivamśapradīpaḥ । jayatu jayatu meghaśyāmlaḥ komalāṅgaḥ । jayatu jayatu kṛṣṇo bhāranāśo mukundaḥ ॥

Victory to the devine son of Devaki, victory to the light of the ancient Vṛśṇi clan, victory to Kṛṣṇa who is like the soft body of a black cloud, victory to the one who lifts the burden (of the earth). Mukunda Mala Strotram vs. 3. Translation: Greg Tebb*

**Kubera**

ओं राजाधिराजाय प्रसह्यसाहिने । नमो वयं वैश्रवनाय कुर्महे । स मे कामान् कामाकामाय मह्यं । कमेश्वारो वैश्रवाणो ददातु । कुबेराय वैश्रवाणाय ।महाराजाय नमः ॥ ओं शान्तिः शान्तिः शान्तिः ॥

Om rājādhirājāya prasahyasāhine । namo vayam vaiśravanāya kurmahe । sa me kāmānkāmakāmāyamahyam । kameśvaro vaiśravāṇo dadātu । kuberāya vaiśravāṇāya । mahārājāya namaḥ ॥ Om śāntiḥ śāntiḥ śāntiḥ ॥

We salute Vaiśravāṇa the king of kings who fulfils all desires. May Lord Vaiśravāṇ the very Lord of desire, fulfil all my many desires. To Lord Kubera Vaiśravāṇa, the great king, salutations. Translation: Rami Śivan

**Navagra Mantra**

ओं नमः सूर्याय चन्द्राय मङ्गलाय बुधाय च ।
गुरुशुक्रशनिभ्याश्च राहुवे केतुवे नमः ॥

Om namaḥ sūryāya candrāya maṅgalāya budhāya ca ।
guruśukraśanibhyāśca rāhuve ketuve nāmaḥ ॥

Salutations to the Sun, the Moon, Mars, and Mercury
And to Jupiter, Venus, Saturn, Rahu and Ketu we salute.

*Translations by Greg Tebb unless otherwise noted.

## CHANTS FROM SHRI SHANKARACHARYA*

### The importance of the teacher

शरीरं सुरूपं तथा वा कलत्रं । यशश्चारु चित्रं धनं मेरुतुल्यं ।
गुरोरंघ्रिपद्मे मनश्चेन लग्नं ततः किं ततः किं ततः किं ततः किं
॥ १ ॥

Śarīram surūpam tathā vā kalatram ı yaśaścāru citram dhanam merutulyam ı guroraṅghripadme manaścena lagnam tataḥ kim tataḥ kim tataḥ kim tataḥ kim ıı 1 ıı

Thy body is well formed, attractive, as also the wife, thy name is prominent and wealth is like Mount Meru. However without adhering to the guidance at the lotus feet of the Guru, what is that? What is that? What is that? What is that? Śrī Śankarācārya, Gurvaṣṭakam. vs. 1

### False Teachers

जटिलो मुण्डी लुञ्छितकेशः काषायाम्बरबहुकृतवेषः ।
पश्यन्नपि च न पश्यति मूढो ह्युदरनिमित्तं बहुकृतवेषः ॥ १४ ॥

Jaṭalo muṇḍī luñchitakeśaḥ kāṣāyāmbarabahukṛtaveṣaḥ ı
paśyannapi ca na paśyati mūḍho hyudaranimittan bahukṛtaveṣaḥ ıı 14

With matted locks, a shaven head, or plucked hair, clad in many ways with ochre-dyed clothes, such fools can see but they do not see (the Truth). They are dressed in these different ways only for the sake of their stomachs (income). Śrī Śankarācārya, Bhaja Govindam. vs. 14

### Samsara

पुनरपि जननं पुनरपि मरणं पुनरपि जननीजठरे शयनम् ।
इह संसारे बहुदुस्तारे कृपयाऽपारे पाहि मुरारे ॥ २१ ॥

Punarapi jananam punarapi maraṇam punarapi jananījaṭhare śayanam ı
iha samsāre bahudustāre kṛpayā'pāre pāhi murāre ıı 21 ıı

Birth again, death again - again to stay in the mother's womb!
Here in this great ocean of Samsara, Oh Murari (Krishna, the slayer of Mura), redeem me through Thy mercy. Śrī Śankarācārya, Bhaja Govindam vs. 21

*This page only.

## Subhashita - Good Sayings

चिन्तयश्च्य चित्तयश्च्ये बिन्दुमत्र विशुश्यते । चिन्त दहति निर्जिवं चित्त दहति जिवनम् ॥ सुभाषित

Cintayaścya chittayaścye bindumatra viśuśyate I cinta dahati nirjivam citta dahati jivanam II Subhaśita

The only (visible) difference between the written words 'funeral pyre' (chinta) & worry (chitta) in the Kanada script is a zero (period). However worry (chitta) burns when you are alive the funeral pyre (chinta) burns when you dead. Translation: Manju Jois

काकाह्वायते काकान् यचिको न तु यचिकान् । काक यचिकोर्मध्ये वरम् काको न तु यचिकः ॥ सुभाषित

Kāka ahvāyate kākān yaciko na tu yachikān I kāka yacikormadhye varam kāko na tu yacikaḥ II Subhaśita

The Kāka (crow) invites his friends to share the food (they find). The Kāka-human being (impudent fellow) invites his friends but stops them from sharing. Translation: Manju Jois

## Prayers Goddess in the hand

कलाग्रे वसते लक्ष्मी कलमध्ये सरस्वती । कलमूल विशालाक्षी प्रभर्ते कलदर्शनम् ॥

Kalāgre vasate lakṣmī kalamadye saraswatī I kalamūle viśālākṣī prabhārte kaladarśanam II

In the morning mediate on the three goddesses in the hand, Lakshmi at the tip of the fingers, Sarasvati in the middle and Vishalakshi at the end of the root/end of the hand.

## Prayer to rise in the morning

उत्तिष्ठोतिष्ठ गोविनद उत्तिष्ठ गरुडध्वज । उत्तिष्ठ कमलकण्ठ त्रैलोक्यं मङ्गलं कुरु ॥ २ ॥

Uttiṣṭhotiṣṭha govinda uttiṣṭha garuḍadhvaja I uttiṣṭha kamalakaṇṭha trilokyam maṅgalam kuru II 2 II

Arise, arise Govinda, arise Garuda, arise the lotus in the throat, may there be auspiciousness in the three worlds. Śrī Venkateśa Suprabhātam vs. 2

### Prayer to step onto the floor in the morning

समुद्रे वसने देवी पर्वतस्तनमण्डले ।
विष्णुपत्नि नमस्तुभ्याम् पादस्पर्शं क्षमस्यमे ॥

Samudre vasne devī parvatastanamaṇḍale । viṣṇupati nastubhyām pādasparśam kṣamasyame ॥

For the Devi, the ocean is her covering, the mountians are her breasts, you who are the consort of Vishnu, please excuse the touch of my feet.

### For Bad dreams

रामस्कन्धं हनुमन्तं वैनतेयं वृकोदरं ।
शयने यः स्मरेन् नित्यं दुःस्वप्नं तस्य नश्यित ॥

Rāmaskandham hanumantam vainateyam vṛkodaram ।
śayane yaḥ smaren nityam duḥswapnam tasya naśyati ॥

Who remembers Rama, Hanuman, Garuda and Bhima at sleep time destroys the bad dreams.

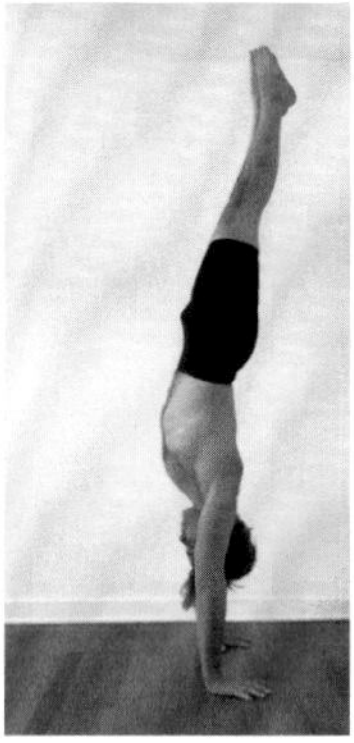
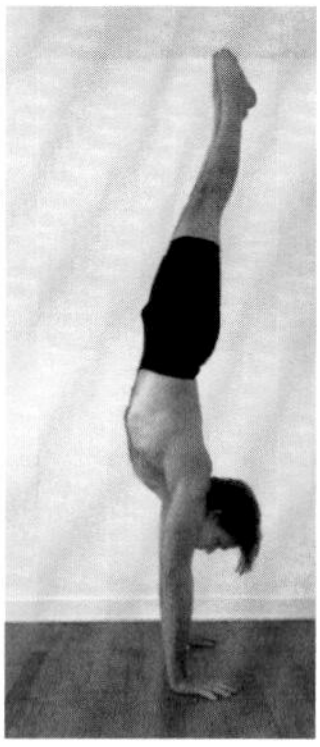

Adho Mukha Vṛkṣāsana
अधो मुख वृक्षासन

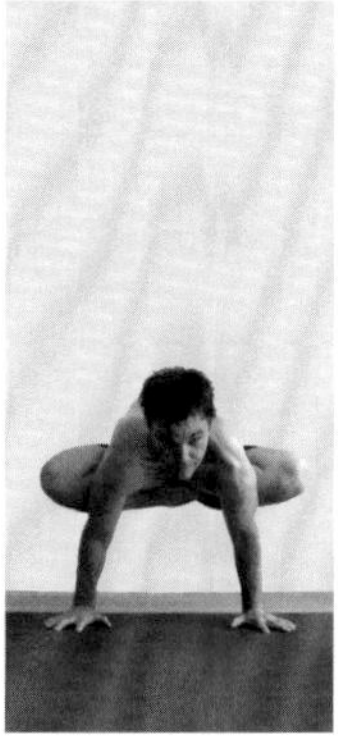

Ūrdhva Kukkuṭāsana
ऊर्ध्व कुक्कुटासन

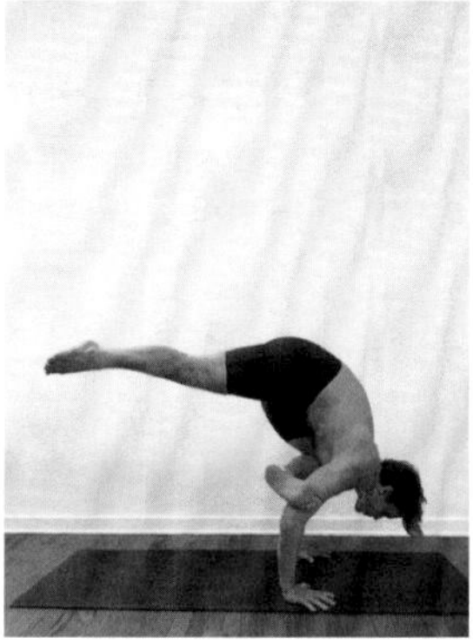

Galavāsana
गलवासन

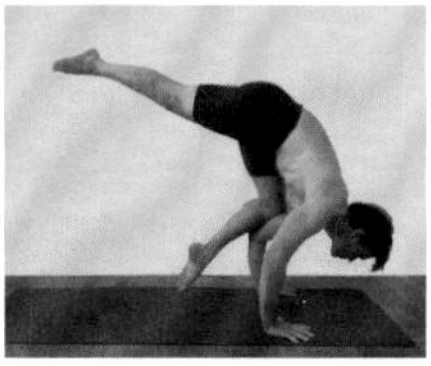

Eka PādaBakāsana
एक पाद बकासन

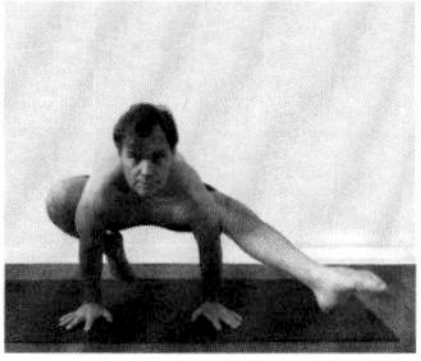

Eka Pāda Bakāsana
एक पाद बकासन

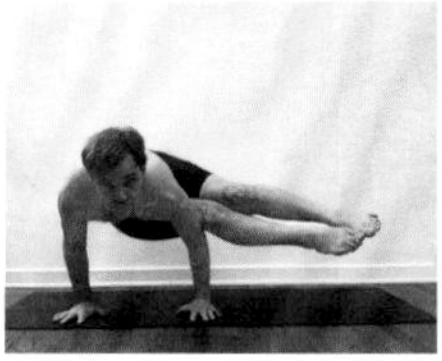

Kauṇḍinyāsana
कौंडिन्यासन

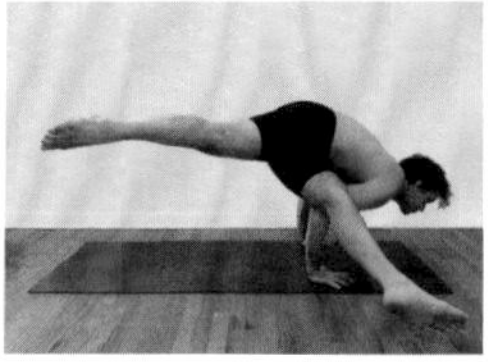

Eka Pāda Kauṇḍinyāsana
एक पाद कौंडिन्यासन

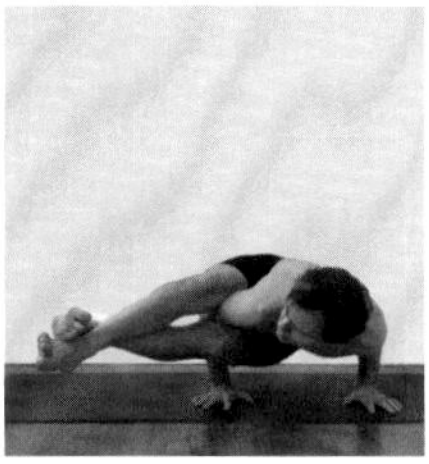

Aṣṭāvakrāsana
अष्टावक्रासन

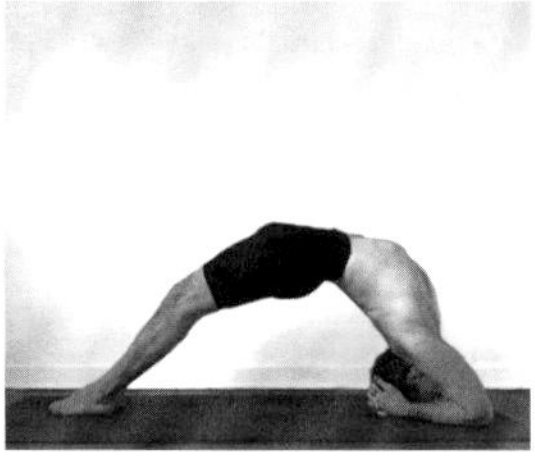

Viparīti Daṇḍāsana
विपरीति दण्डासन

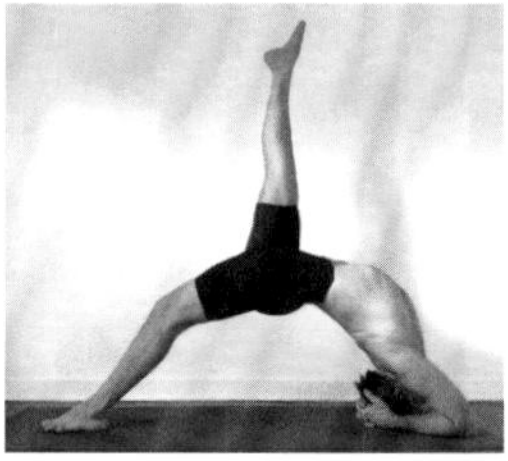

Eka Pāda Viparīti Daṇḍāsana
एक पाद विपरीति दण्डासन

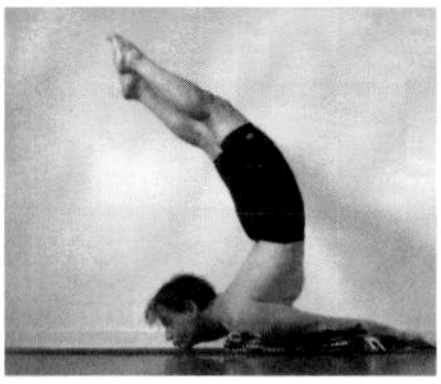

Viparīti Śalabhāsana
विपरीति शलभासन

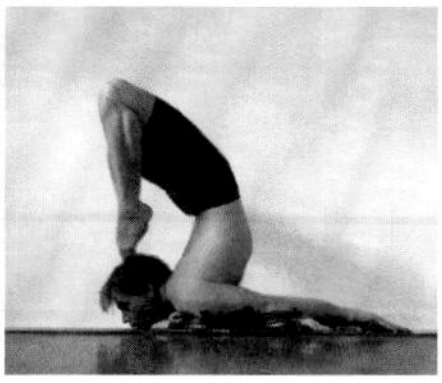

Viparīti Śalabhāsana
विपरीति शलभासन

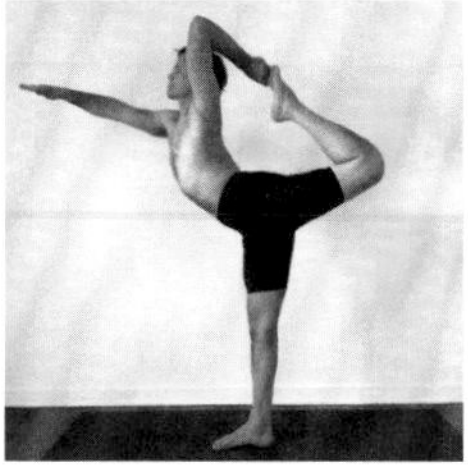

Naṭarājāsana
नटराजासन

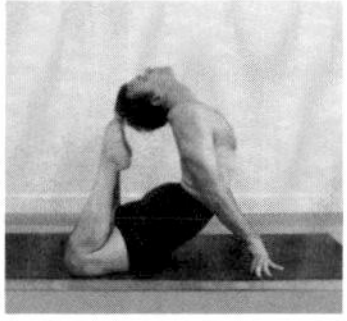

Rāja Kapotāsana
राज कपोतासन

SECOND FROM RIGHT: JETT ULANER SARACHEK

## Diacritical marks

| | |
|---|---|
| ā | long vowel, as in father |
| ī | police |
| ū | prude |
| ṛ | 'ri' |
| k | kill, seek |
| c | 'ch', chapel |
| ch | 'chh', churchill |
| e | bet |
| ṅ | sing |
| ñ | singe |
| ṇ | none |
| ṭ | true |
| ṭh | anthill |
| ḍ | drum |
| ḍh | redhaired |
| ś | sure |
| ṣ | shun, bush |
| ḥ | 'hih', Visarga, (stopping the breath) |

## Sanskṛit pronunciation guide

VOWELS

अ a, आ ā, इ i, ई ī, उ u, ऊ ū, ऋ ṛ, ॠ ṝ,
ऌ ḷ, ॡ ḹ, ए e, ऐ ai, ओ o, औ au, अं aṁ, अः aḥ,

CONSONANTS

क ka, ख kha, ग ga, ख gha, ङ ṅa, च ca, छ ca, ज ja, झ jha, ञ ña,
ट ṭa, ठ ṭha, ड ḍa, ढ ḍha, ण ṇa, त ta, थ tha, द da, ध dha, न na,
प pa, फ pha , ब ba, भ bha, म ma,
य ya, र ra, ल la, व va (wa) श śa, ष ṣa, स sa, ह ha

NUMERALS

1 १ एकं ekam
2 २ द्वे dve
3 ३ त्रीणि trīṇi
4 ४ चत्वारि catvāri
5 ५ पञ्च pañca
6 ६ षत् ṣat
7 ७ सप्त sapta
8 ८ अष्टौ aṣṭau
9 ९ नव nava
10 १० दश daśa
11 ११ एकादश ekādaśa
12 १२ द्वादश dvādaśa
13 १३ त्रयोदश trayodaśa
14 १४ चतुर्दश caturdaśa
15 १५ पञ्चदश pañcadaśa
16 १६ षोदश ṣodaśa
17 १७ सप्तदश saptadaśa
0 ० शुञ्य śuñya

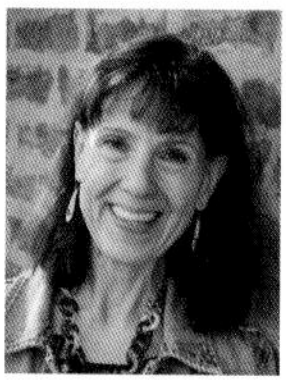

**Christine Fish Moulton** is a professional musician and associate professor of flute at Mansfield University of PA. She has been practicing Ashtanga Yoga for over 20 years.

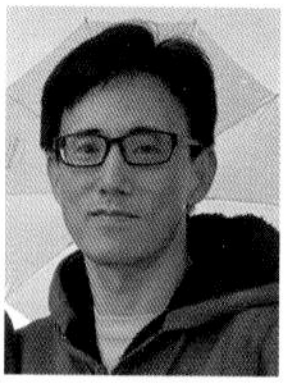

**Benety Goh** lives in New Jersey with his wife Shirley and daughter Evelyn. He is a long time Ashtanga Yoga practitioner.

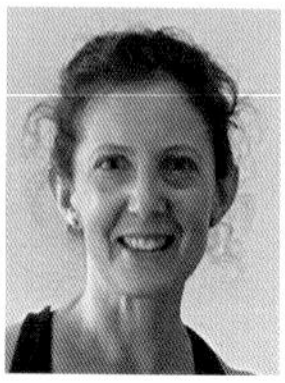

**Nicole Cohen** lives in NYC with her husband and four children. She is the proud mother of two sets of twins and works as a learning specialist. Her Ashtanga Yoga practice plays a vital role in helping her maintain health and wellness during her extremely busy days.

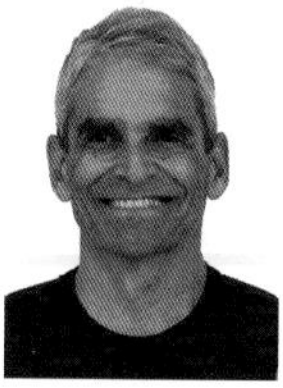

**Erik Marrero** found yoga in the Spring of 2007. As a Stage IV cancer patient with severe osteoporosis, he started practicing yoga to deal with the side effects of these conditions and medications. After 10 years of practicing yoga therapy daily, Erik's Stage IV cancer was completely gone, and his severe osteoporosis completely reversed. Erik is grateful to have been introduced to this healing practice. He has been a long term student of Manju Jois and lives in southern New Jersey with his wife Debbie.

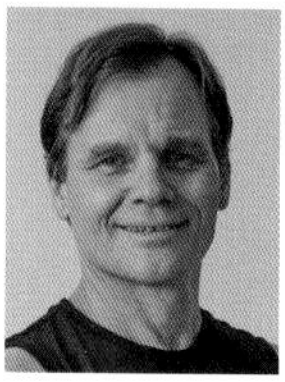

**Greg Tebb** first discovered Ashtanga Yoga in 1986 as a teenager in New Zealand. He was a professional dancer and martial arts instructor before teaching yoga. Greg has apprenticed and assisted Manju Jois since 2000. He co-authored two training manuals with Manju before this book.

Thanks to all of the models for thier hard work and thanks to Mandy at Juluka Yoga School in Hillsdale, NJ.

**Āsana:** position, pose
**Adho:** downward
**Adho Mukha Śvānāsana:** downward facing dog position, used during sun salutation and jump backs (ṣat)
**Agra:** foremost, preeminent, prominent point, tip
**Aṅga:** limb
**Aṅguṣṭa:** thumb
**Antara:** inside
**Antara dṛṣṭi:** closing eyes and looking in
**Antarikṣa/ūrdhva:** sky/upward
**Antarikṣa dṛṣṭi:** sky gazing, gazing upward
**Ardha:** half
**Ardha Baddha Padmottanāsana:** half bound intense leg position
**Ardha Baddha Padma Paścimatānāsana:** half bound lotus, extended back of body position
**Ardha Candrāsana:** half moon position
**Ardha Matysendrāsana:** pose of Matsyendra
**Ashtanga:** (aṣṭāṅga) the eight limbed system of sage Patañjali; name of the Jois family yoga system
**Aṣṭau:** 8
**Aṣṭāvakrāsana:** pose of Aṣṭāvakra
**Aṣṭāvakra:** a brahman sage. 'Eight crooks', son of the sage Kahoḍa. While in the womb Aṣṭāvakra was disturbed by his father's scholarly lack of attention for his mother. Upset Kahoḍa cursed his son to be born crippled. Later Aṣṭāvakra saved his father, who had drowned. Kahoḍa being pleased, relieved his son of his crookedness by directing him to bathe in the Samaṅga river.
**Ayāma:** control

**Baddha:** bound
**Baddha Hasta Śīrṣāsana:** bound hand head position
**Baddha Koṇāsana:** bound angle pose
**Baddha Padmāsana:** Bound lotus position
**Baka:** crane
**Bakāsana:** crane position
**Bala:** child
**Balāsana:** child position
**Bandha:** lock, bound
**Bhāga:** part, section, e.g. 'left side of an asana'
**Bhairava:** "the terrible" aspect of Śiva
**Bhairavī:** "the terrible" aspect of Parvatī
**Bhairava/Bhairavī Mudrā:** seal of Rudra/Rudrānī
**Bhairavāsana:** pose of Bhairava
**Bhairava:** name of sage, 'terrible, frightful, formidable', a form of Śiva.
**Bharadvāja:** name of sage
**Bharadvājāsana:** position of Bharadvāja
**Bheka:** frog
**Bhekāsana:** frog position
**Bhuja:** arm
**Bhujapīdāsana:** pressure the arm position
**Brū:** eyebrow
**Brūmadya dṛṣṭi:** eyebrow centre gazing

**Cakra:** *chakra*, wheel
**Catur:** four
**Caturdaśa:** 14
**Caturtha:** 4th
**Caturtha Baddha Hasta Śīrṣāsana:** fourth bound-hand head position
**Caturaṅga Dañḍāsana:** Four limbed rod position used in the sun:salutation and jump: backs (Catwāri)
**Catwāri:** 4
**Cikitsā:** administering remedies, curing, healing Cin (cit): to perceive, observe
**Cin Mudrā:** observing mudra
**Cakorāsana:** pose of Cakora (Chakora).
**Cakora (Chakora):** a greek partridge, said to be nourished by moon beams.

**Dakṣina:** right/south
**Daṇḍa:** rod, stick
**Daṇḍāsana:** rod position
**Daśa:** 10
**Dhanur:** bow
**Dhanurāsana:** bow position
**Dig:** point, direction
**Digāsana:** pointing posture. From the Sanskṛt root 'diś' to point.
**Dīrgha:** long
**Dūrvasāsana:** pose of pose of Dūrvāsās, 'naked, badly clothed', devotee/incarnation of Śiva, known for his quick temper.
**Dwādaśa:** 12
**Dwe:** 2
**Dwitīya:** 2nd
**Dwitīya Baddha Hasta Śīrṣāsana:** second bound-hand head position
**Dwitīya Mukta Hasta Śīrṣāsana:** second liberated-hand head position
**Dwe Pāda Śīrṣāsana:** two feet (behind) head position (Dwe: 2)
**Dṛṣṭi:** drishti, gaze point; there are 10 Dṛṣṭi's used in this book. Nasāgra (nose tip) the most commonly used, Pādāṅguṣṭha (big toe), hastāgra (end point of hand), Nabhi (navel), Bhūmadhi (the place over/above the eyebrow) also called Brūmadya, Pārśva (the side), Antara (inside), Ūrdhva (upward) also called Antarikṣa (sky, 'place between heaven & earth'). All are meditation points. They focus the mind, stimulate the subtle energy, and correct the subtle alignment of the body.

**Eka:** 1
**Eka Pāda Śīrṣāsana:** one foot (behind) head position
**Ekādaśa:** 11
**Ekam:** 1

**Gālavāsana:** pose of Gālava.
**Gālava:** pupil of Viśvāmitra, sanskṛt grammarian, author of Dharma Śāstra
**Garbha:** Womb
**Garbhapiṇḍāsana:** round the womb position
**Go:** cow
**Gomukhāsana:** cow face position

**Hala:** plough
**Halāsana:** plough position

**Hanumanāsana:** pose of Hanuman, monkey king, hero of the Rāmāyaṇa, devotee of Rāma
**Hasta:** hand
**Hastāgra dṛṣṭi:** end of finger gazing

**Jānu:** knee
**Jānu Śīrṣāsana:** head to knee pose

**Kapota:** dove, pigeon
**Kapotāsana:** dove position
**Karanī:** doing, making
**Karṇa:** ear
**Karṇapīḍāsana:** ear pressure position
**Kauṇḍinyāsana:** pose of Kauṇḍinya
**Kauṇḍinya:** a sanskṛt scholar and poet, known for his expertise in Vyākarana sanskṛt grammar and logistics. Also known as Jayadeva author of Gita Govinda.
**Kśyapāsana:** pose of Kśyapa
**Kśyapa:** name of a sage, 'having black teeth', author hymns in Rig Veda, descendant of Marīcī.
**Kāraṇḍava:** Himālayan duck
**Kāraṇḍavāsana:** Himālayan duck position (ref: Maha bharata 4:30:31)
**Koṇa:** angle
**Krauñca:** heron
**Krauñcāsana:** heron position
**Kukkuṭa:** rooster
**Kukkuṭāsana:** rooster position
**Kūrma:** turtle, second incarnation of Vishnu
**Kūrmāsana:** turtle position

**Laghu:** light, quick
**Laghu Vajrāsana:** light thunderbolt position

**Madya:** middle
**Matsya:** Fish, incarnation of Viṣṇu, saviour of Manu and the Vedas
**Matsyāsana:** fish position
**Matsyendra:** name of famous haṭha yogi
**Matsyendrāsana:** pose of Matsyendra
**Marīci (Marīca):** ray of light, name of Prajāpati (father of the creatures), attendant to Sūrya.
**Marīcyāsana:** position of Marīci (Marīcāsana)
**Marma:** a medicinal/meditation point used in Ayurvedic medicine and yoga
**Mayūra:** peacock
**Mayūrāsana:** peacock position
**Meridian:** or Nadī, a pathway in the body. They carry subtle energy through the body.
**Mukha:** face Mukta, liberated
**Mudrā:** seal
**Mūla:** root
**Mūla bandha:** root lock

**Nabhi:** navel
**Nabhi dṛṣṭi:** navel gazing

**Nadī:** river
**Nadī Shodhana:** river (in body) cleaning

**Nakra:** crocodile
**Nakrāsana:** crocodile position
**Namaskāraḥ:** salutation
**Nava:** 9
**Nāsā:** nose
**Nasāgra dṛṣṭi:** preeminent nose gaze (end of nose)
**Naṭarājāsana:** pose of Naṭarāja
**Naṭarāja:** epitaph for Śiva. 'dance king', King of the dance, movement, Āsanas.
**Nāva:** boat
**Nāvāsana:** boat position
**Nidra:** sleep

**Padma:** lotus
**Pañca:** 5
**Pañcadaśa:**15
**Pari:** rotated
**Parigha:** iron or wooden beam, bar (used for shutting a gate)
**Parighāsana:** bar (for gate) position
**Parivṛtta Pārśva Koṇāsana:** rotated side angle pose
**Parivṛtta Trikoṇāsana:** rotated 3 angle position
**Parvata:** mountain
**Parvatāsana:** mountain position
**Paścima:** back of body, west
**Paścimatānāsana:** extended back of body position
**Pāda:** foot, leg
**Pādahastāsana:** hand foot position
**Pādāṅguṣṭhāsana:** big toe position
**Pādāṅguṣṭhāsana dṛṣṭi:** gazing big toe
**Pārśva:** side
**Pārśva Dhanurāsana:** side bow position
**Pārśva dṛṣṭi:** side gazing
**Pārśva Koṇāsana:** side angle position
**Pārśvottānāsana:** side lengthened position
**Pāśa:** noose
**Pāśāsana:** noose position
**Piccha:** feathered, (pronounced "pincha")
**Piccha Mayūrāsana:** feathered peacock position
**Piṇḍa:** solid, compact, a round mass
**Piṇḍāsana:** round position
**Pīḍā:** pressure, squeeze
**Prasārita:** spread apart
**Prasārita Padotānāsana:** feet spread apart lengthened leg stretch
**Prathama:** first
**Prathama Baddha Hasta Śīrṣāsana:** first bound-hand head position
**Prathama Mukta Hasta Śīrṣāsana:** first liberated-hand head position
**Prāṇa:** energy
**Prāṇāyāma:** (prāṇa-āyama) breath control. Ancient exercises developed to energize the body for health and meditation. It stabilizes the five airs in the body: Prāṇa (heart), Apāna (tailbone), Samāna (navel), Udāna (throat) Vyāna (limbs & outside body).

**Pūraka:** inhale
**Pūrva:** front, east, first, prominent
**Pūrvatānāsana:** extended front of the body position

**Recaka:** exhale
**Roga:** disease, sickness

**Sama:** same/equal
**Samasthitiḥ:** equal standing or remaining position
**Sapta:** 7
**Saptadaśa:** 17
**Sarva:** all
**Sarvāṅgāsana:** all limb position
**Setu:** bridge
**Setu Bandhāsana:** bridge bound position
**Skanda:** name of sage Kārtikeya god of war,'leaping, quicksilver'
**Skandāsana:** pose of Skanda
**Śalabha:** locust
**Śalabhāsana:** locust position
**Ṣat:** 6
**Śava:** corpse
**Śavāsāna:** corpse position
**Śīrṣa:** head
**Śīrṣāsana:** headstand
**Śloka:** pronounced shloka, a 'sanskṛt teaching', a sanskṛt verse in the Anuṣṭup metre, the most common meter in the sanskṛt language
**Ṣodaśa:** 16
**Śodhana:** cleaning (from *śundh*, pure)
**Sthitiḥ:** standing, remaining
**Supta:** sleeping, reclining, supine
**Supta Koṇāsana:** sleeping angle pose
**Supta Kūrmāsana:** sleeping turtle position
**Supta Ūrdhva Pāda Vajrāsana:** reclining upward facing leg thunderbolt pose
**Supta Vajrāsana:** sleeping thunderbolt position
**Sūrya:** sun
**Śvāna:** dog

**Tān:** to stretch, extend
**Titibha:** firefly, Daitya son of Kaśyapa
**Titibhāsana:** firefly position
**Tri:** 3
**Tiryañc:** obliquely crookedly
**Tiryañc Mukhaika Pāda Paścimatānāsana:** one limb obliquely facing extended back of body position
**Tṛtīya:** 3rd
**Tṛtīya Baddha Hasta Śīrṣāsana:** third bound-hand head position
**Tṛtīya Mukta Hasta Śīrṣāsana:** third liberated-hand head position
**Trivikramāsana:** pose of Trivikrama
**Trivikrama:** epitaph for Viṣṇu, 'three steps' uninterrupted, one who strides through the three worlds. Also the name of the son of Vyāsa (author Maha Bhārata).
**Triyodaśa:** 13
**Trīṇi:** 3

**Ubhaya (Ubhayā):** both
**Ubhaya Pādāṅguṣṭhāsana:** both feet big toe position
**Uddiyāna:** upward flying
**Uddiyāna bandha:** upward flying lock
**Ujjāyī Prāṇāyāma:** Victorious energy control. This is a traditional prāṇāyāma technique, one of the 8 kumbhakas: sūryabhedam, *ujjāyī*, sītkārī, śītalī, bhastrikā, bhrāmarī, mūrchā and plāvinī. HYP (Haṭha Yoga Pradīpikā) 2:44.
It is the breath technique used in the Aṣṭāṅga yoga system. A deep sound breath, equal on the inhale and exhale, continuously performed from the first sun salutation until finished.

'mukham samyamya nāḍībhyāmākṛṣya pavanam śanaiḥ / yathā lagati kaṇṭhāttu hṛdayāvadhi sasvanam' HYP 2:52.
"Breathe the air slowly through both nostrils, adhering (feeling) it in the throat up into the chest," and then out both nostrils again with sound.

'ślemadaṣaharam kanṭhe dehānalivardhanam';
"This prāṇāyāma helps remove problems caused by phlegm in the throat and increases the digestive fire in the body.";

'nāḍījalodarādhātugatadoṣavināṣanam / jacchatā tiṣṭhatākāryamujāyyākhyam tu kumbhakam' HYP 2:53
"This prāṇāyāma called Ujjāyī removes issues from the body channels: (meridians), excess fluid in the tissue (dropsy) and rebalances the Dośas (kapha, pitta, vāta). It can be done moving or sitting."

**Utkaṭa:** fierce, powerful
**Utkaṭāsana:** powerful position
**Uttāna:** stretched out, expanded
**Uttāna Pādāsana:** intense leg stretch position
**Utthita:** extended, standing, rising, risen
**Utthita Hasta Pādāṅguṣṭhāsana:** extended hand big toe position
**Utthita Trikoṇāsana:** three angle extended position
**Utpluta:** jump up, spring upon suddenly
**Utplutiḥ:** lifting and holding position
**Upa:** (prefix) down, close to, near, by the side
**Upaviṣṭha Koṇasana:** spread in front of the seat position
**Ūrdhva:** upright, rising or tending upward
**Ūrdhva Mukha Paścimatānāsana:** upward facing back extended position
**Uṣṭra:** camel
**Uṣṭrāsana:** camel position
**Ūrdhva:** upward
**Ūrdhva Dhanurāsana:** upward bow position
**Ūrdhva Mukha Śvānāsana:** upward facing dog position, used in jump backs and sun salutation (pañca)
**Ūrdhva Padmāsana:** upward lotus position
**Vajra:** thunderbolt
**Vaśiṣṭhāsana:** pose of Vaśiṣṭha
**Vaśiṣṭha:** name of a sage, alternate spelling Vasiṣṭha, 'most excellent, best', rival of Viśvāmitra. Owner of Nandīni the 'cow of plenty', author of Yoga Vasiṣṭha and texts on the Law and Vedic literature.
**Vātāyana:** horse
**Vātāyanāsana:** horse position

**Vinyāsa:** breathing system, 'moving in and out of asana'
**Virañcāsana:** pose of Virañcā
**Virañcā:** name of Brahma, the quality of expansion in the Guṇa Trinity
**Viṣṇu:** Śiva
**Viś:** to spread, extend, pervade
**Viśvāmitrāsana:** pose of Viśvāmitra
**Viśvāmitra:** name of sage, 'viśvā-mitra' (universal-friend), an ancient sage said to have meditated for 1000 years in Himālayas, and aquired heavenly powers. Closely associated with, and an antagonist to the sage Vaśiṣṭha.
**Vīra:** heroic, brave man
**Vīrabhadra:** hero greeted by Śiva out of his matted hair
**Vīrabhadrāsana:** Warrior (hero Vīrabhradra) pose
**Viparīta:** Inverted
**Viparīta Karaṇī:** Making inverted (position)
**Vṛtta:** modification, occurred, a round, circular

**Wama:** left side, north

**Yoga:** yoke
**Yoga/Roga Cikitsā:** yoking/disease curing
**Yoga Nidrāsana:** yoga sleep position

## Bibliography

**Hatha Yoga Pradipika**
Commentary Swami Vishnu-Devananda
Motilal Barnarsidass Publishers Private Limited, Delhi; OM Lotus Publications, 1987

Dr M.A. Jayashree, Anantha Research Foundation
384 Krishna Vilas Road, Mysore-570024, India, 2006

**Gheranda Samhita**
Edited Swami Digambarji & Dr M.L. Gharote
Published by Shri O.P. Tiwari, Secretary, for the Kailvalyadharma, S.M.Y.M., Lonavia, Maharashtra, India, 1997

The Original Sanskrit and an English Translation
James Mallinson, YogaVidya.com, Woodstock, NY, 2004

**Nathamuni's Yoga Rajasya** Translated by TKV Desikachar
Krishnamacharya Yoga Mandiram, 31, 4th Cross Street, R K Nagar, Chennai - 600028, India, 2010

**Chinese Acupuncture and Moxibustion** Chief Editor by Cheng Xinnong
Foreign Language Press, 24 Baiwanzhuang Road, Beijing 100037, China, 1999

**Anatomy Trains** 2nd Edition Thomas W. Meyers
Published by Sarena Wolfaard, Churchill Livingstone-ELSEVIER, 2009

**Ashtanga Yoga Workshop with Manju Jois** DVD Manju Jois and Wolvington Productions 2006

**Yoga Kosha** Kaivalyadhama S.M.Y.M. Samiti, Lonavla, Dist. Pune, Maharashtra

**Light on Yoga** BKS Iyengar: George Allen & Unwin Ltd, 1968

**The Yoga Tradition** Georg Feuerstein: Hohm Press, Arizona

**Yoga Mala** K. Pattabhi Jois; published by Eddie Stern/Patanjali Yoga Shala, New York, NY, 1999

**Mantra Pushpam** The President, Ramakrishna Math, Khar, Mumbai-400 052

"Deliver the message that it is about self-practice, 'become one with yourself' that is what yoga is about."

Manju Jois

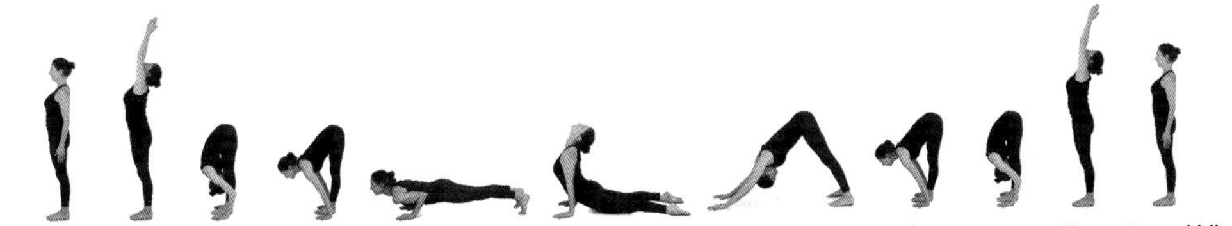

Samasthitiḥ Ekam Dwe Trīṇi Catvāri Pañca Ṣat Sapta Aṣṭau Nava Samasthitiḥ

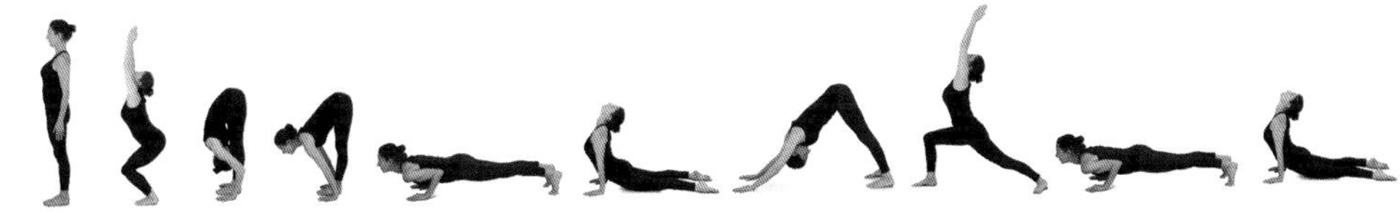

Samasthitiḥ Ekam Dwe Trīṇi Catvāri Pañca Ṣat Sapta Aṣṭau Nava

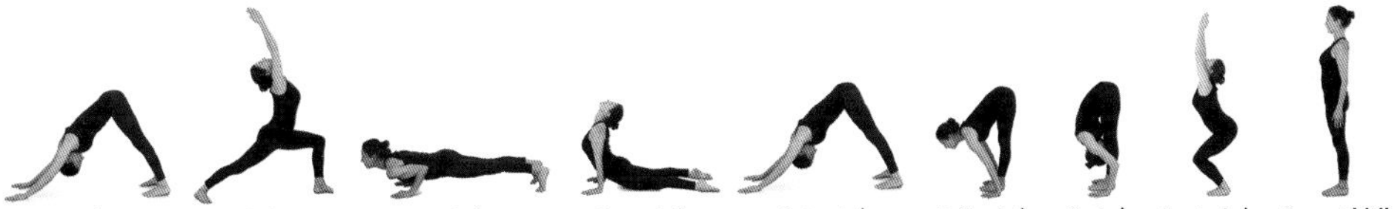

Daśa Ekādaśa (left leg foward) Dvādaśa Trayodaśa Caturdaśa Pañcadaśa Ṣodaśa Saptadaśa Samasthitiḥ

## Standing Poses

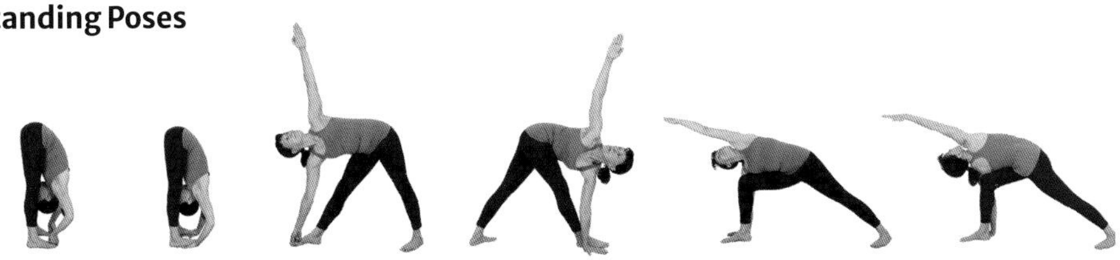

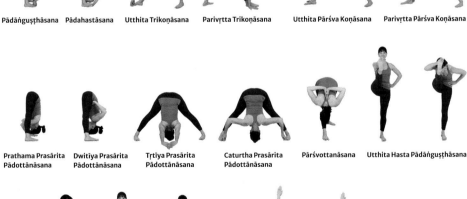

Pādāṅguṣṭhāsana Pādahastāsana Utthita Trikoṇāsana Parivṛtta Trikoṇāsana Utthita Pārśva Koṇāsana Parivṛtta Pārśva Koṇāsana

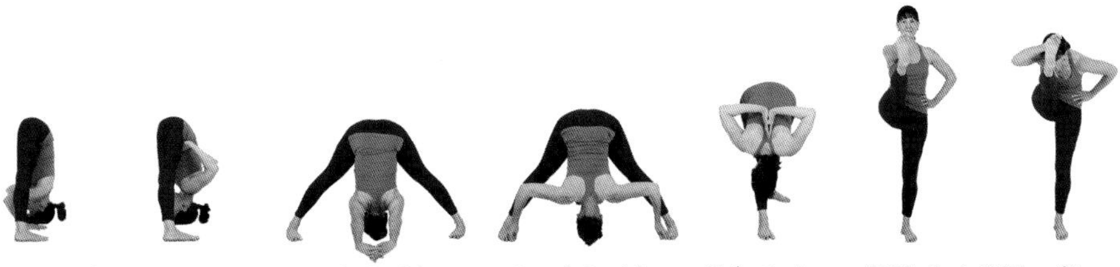

Prathama Prasārita Pādottānāsana Dwitīya Prasārita Pādottānāsana Tṛtīya Prasārita Pādottānāsana Caturtha Prasārita Pādottānāsana Pārśvottanāsana Utthita Hasta Pādāṅguṣṭhāsana

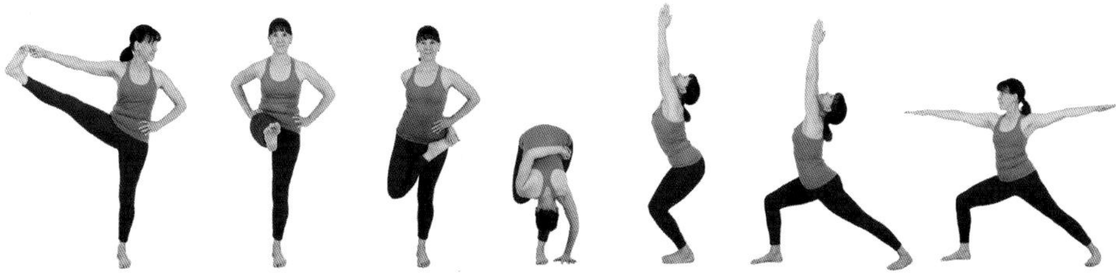

Utthita Hasta Pādāṅguṣṭhāsana Ardha Baddha Padmottānāsana Utkaṭāsana Vīrabhadrāsana Vīrabhadrāsana

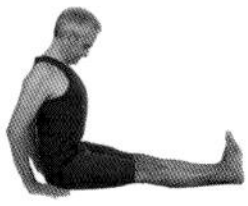
Daṇḍāsana

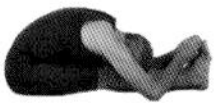
Prathama Paścimatānāsana

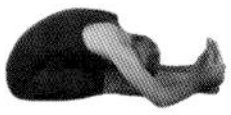
Dwitīya Paścimatānāsana

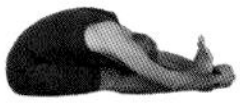
Tṛtīya Paścimatānāsana

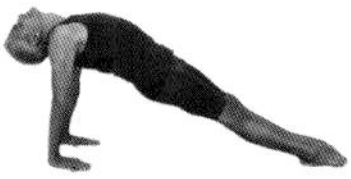
Pūrvatānāsanam

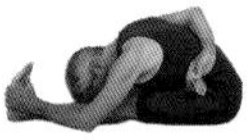
Ardha Baddha Padma Paścimatānāsana

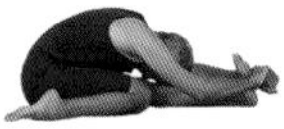
Tiryañc Mukhaika Pāda Paścimatānāsana

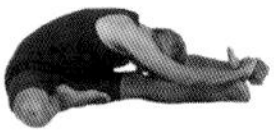
Prathama Jānu Śīrṣāsana

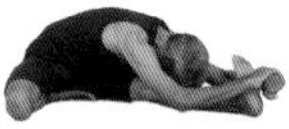
Dwitīya Jānu Śīrṣāsana

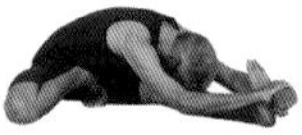
Tṛtīya Jānu Śīrṣāsana

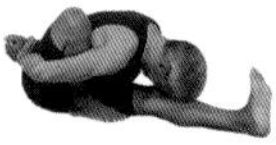
Prathama Marīcyāsana

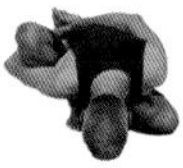
Dwitīya Marīcyāsana

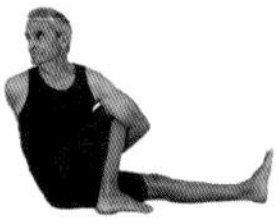
Tṛtīya Marīcyāsana

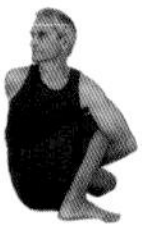
Caturtha Marīcyāsana

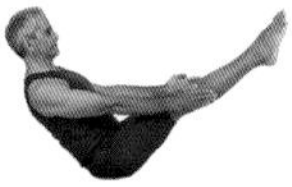
Nāvāsana

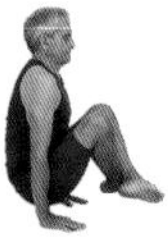
Utplutiḥ

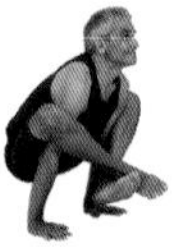
Bhujapīḍāsana

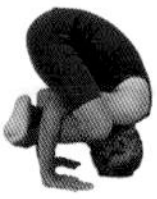
Bhujapīḍāsana

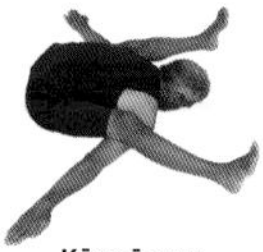
Kūrmāsana

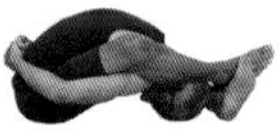
Supta Kūrmāsana

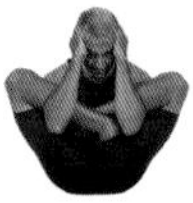
Garbhapiṇḍāsana

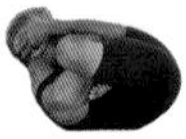
Garbhapiṇḍāsana

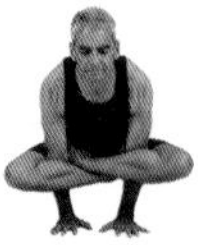
Kukkuṭāsana

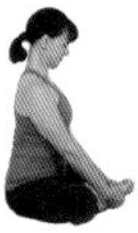
Baddha Koṇāsana

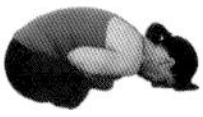
Prathama Baddha Koṇāsana

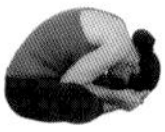
Dwitīya Baddha Koṇāsana

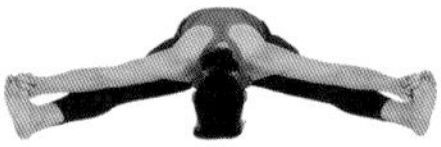
Upaviṣṭha Koṇāsana

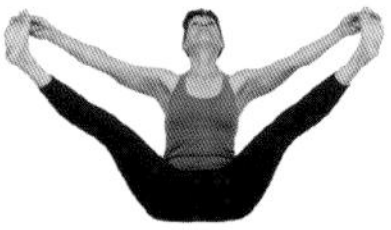
Ūrdhva Mukha Upaviṣṭha Koṇāsana

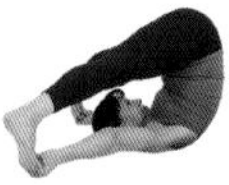
Supta Koṇāsana

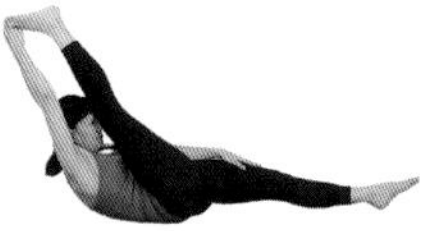
Supta Pādāṅguṣṭhāsana

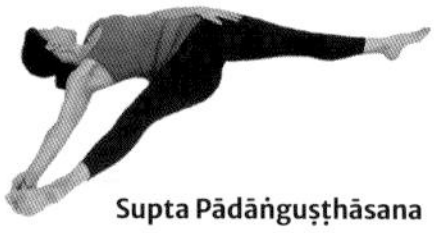
Supta Pādāṅguṣṭhāsana

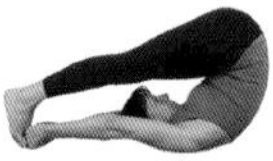
Ubhaya Pādāṅguṣṭhāsana

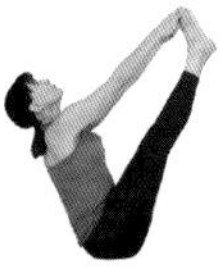
Ūrdhva Pādāṅguṣṭhāsana

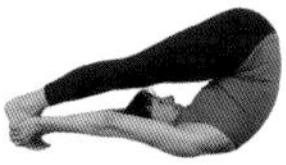
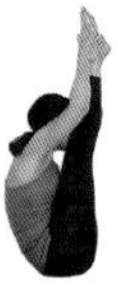
Ūrdhva Mukha Paścimatānāsana

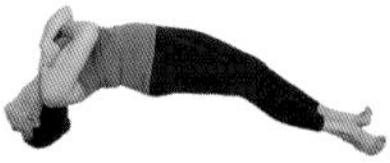
Setu Bandhāsana

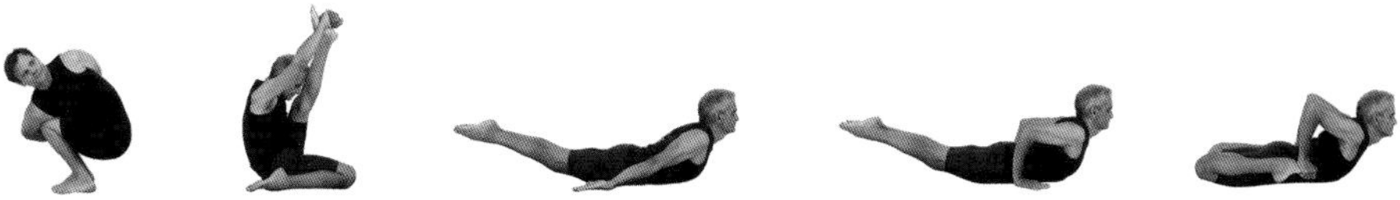

Pāśāsana | Krauñcāsana | Prathama Śalabhāsana | Dwitīya Śalabhāsana | Bhekāsana

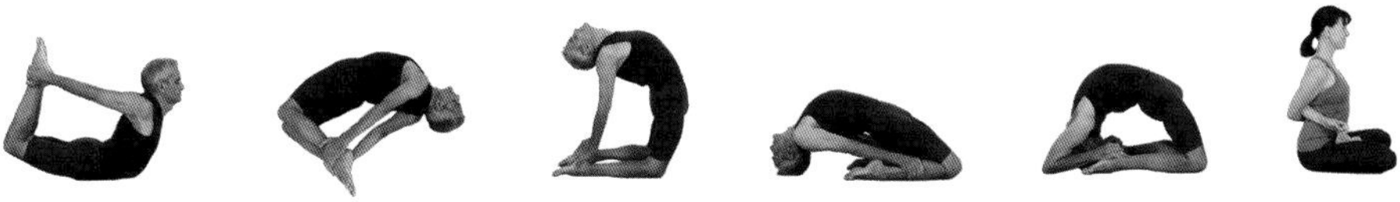

Dhanurāsana | Pārśva Dhanurāsana | Uṣṭrāsana | Laghu Vajrāsana | Kapotāsana | Supta Vajrāsana

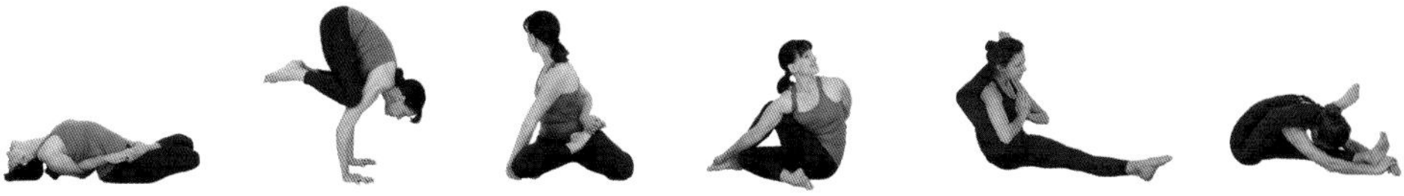

Supta Vajrāsana | Prathama Bakāsana Dwitīya Bakāsana | Bharadvājāsana | Ardha Matysendrāsana | Eka Pāda Śīrṣāsana | Eka Pāda Śīrṣāsana

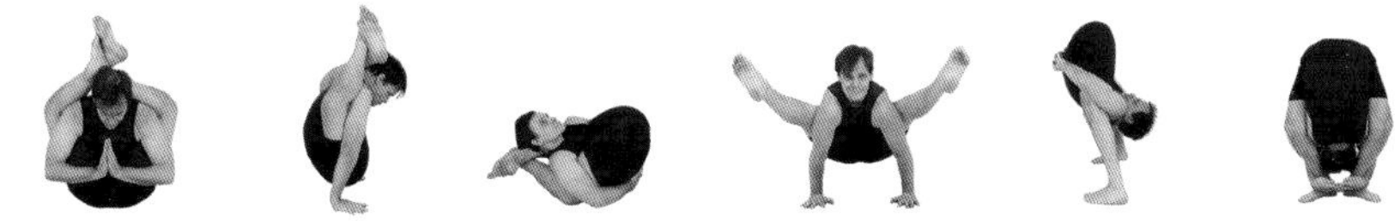

Dwi Pāda Śīrṣāsana | Utplutiḥ | Yoga Nidrāsana | Titibhāsana | Titibhāsana | Titibhāsana

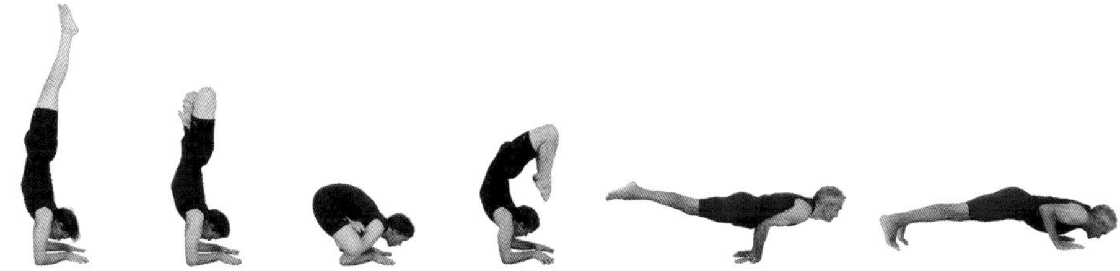

Piccha Mayūrāsana | Kāraṇḍavāsana | Kāraṇḍavāsana | Vṛścikāsana | Mayūrāsana | Nakrāsana

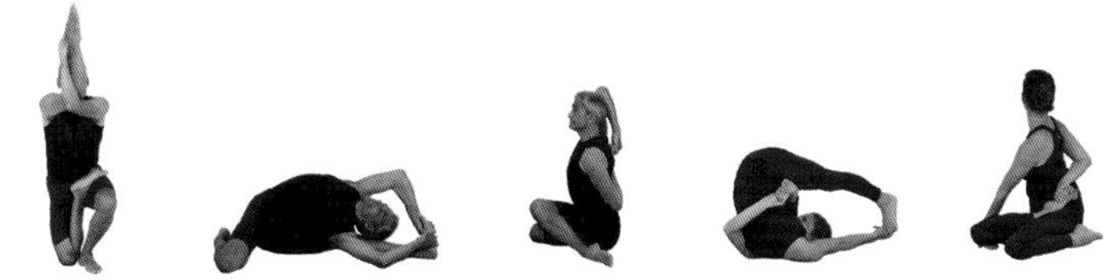

Vatayanāsana | Parighāsana | Gomukhāsana | Supta Ūrdhva Pāda Vajrāsana

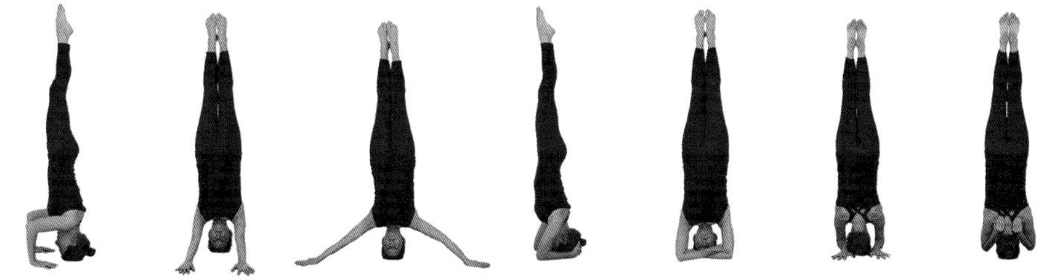

Prathama Mukta Hasta Śīrṣāsana | Dwitīya Mukta Hasta Śīrṣāsana | Tṛtīya Mukta Hasta Śīrṣāsana | Prathama Baddha Hasta Śīrṣāsana | Dwitīya Baddha Hasta Śīrṣāsana | Tṛtīya Baddha Hasta Śīrṣāsana | Cathurta Baddha Hasta Śīrṣāsana

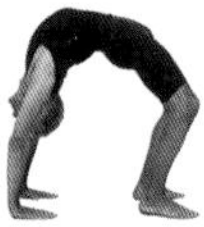

Ūrdhva Dhanurāsana

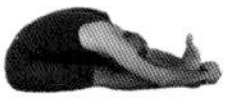

Tṛtīya Paścimatānāsana

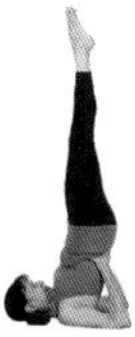

Sarvāṅgāsana

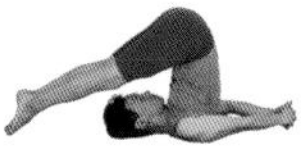

Halāsana

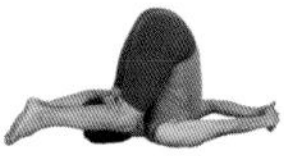

Karṇapīḍāsana

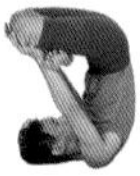

Ūrdhva Padmāsana

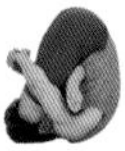

Piṇḍāsana

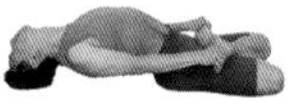

Matsyāsana

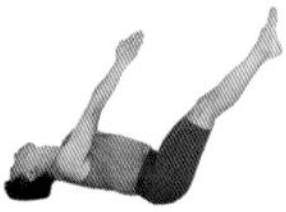

Uttāna Pādāsana

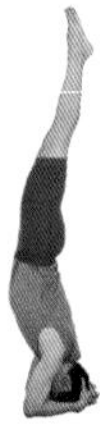

Baddha Hasta Śīrṣāsana

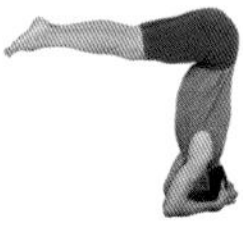

Ardha Candrāsana

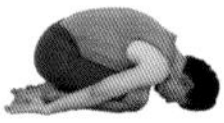

Balāsana

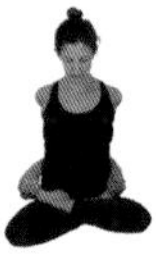

Baddha Padmāsana

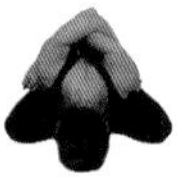

Yoga Mudrā

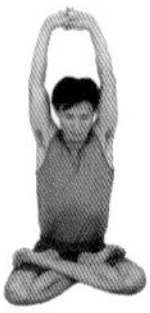

Parvatāsana

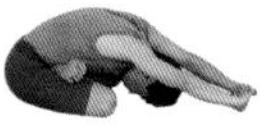

Parvatāsana

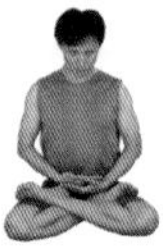

Bhairava/Bhairavī Mudrā

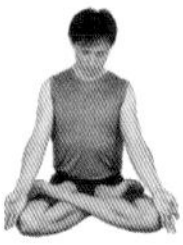

Cin Mudrā

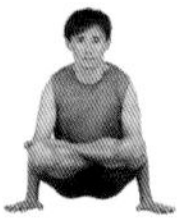

Utplutiḥ

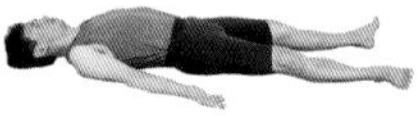

Śavasāna

## Shanti Mantra

Om saha nāvavatu | saha nau bhunaktu |
saha vīryam karavāvahai |
tejasvināvadhītamastu mā vidviṣāvahai ||
om śāntiḥ śāntiḥ śāntiḥ ||

Om śan no mitraḥ śam varuṇaḥ ı śan no bhavatvaryamā ı śan na indro bṛhaspatiḥ ı śan no viṣnururukramaḥ ı namo brahmaṇe ı namaste vāyo ı tvameva pratyakṣam brahmāsi ı tvāmeva pratyakṣam brahma vadiṣyāmi ı ṛtam vadiṣyāmi ı satyam vadiṣyāmi ı tanmāmavatu ı tadvaktāramavatu ı avatu mām ı avatu vaktāram ıı Om śāntiḥ śāntiḥ śāntiḥ ıı

Om bhadram karṇebhiḥ śṛṇuyāma devāḥ ı bhadram paśyemākṣbhiryajatrāḥ ı sthirairaṅgaistuṣṭuvāgamsastanūbhiḥ ı vyaśema devahitaṁ yadāyuḥ ı swasti na indro vrddhaśravāḥ ı swasti naḥ pūṣā viśvavedāḥ ı swasti no tārkṣyo ariṣṭanemiḥ ı swasti no bṛhaspatirdadhātu ıı Om śāntiḥ śāntiḥ śāntiḥ ıı

Om namo brahmaṇe namo astvagnaye namaḥ pṛthivyai nama oṣadhībhyaḥ ı namo vāce namo vācaspataye namo viṣṇave bṛhate karomi ıı Om śāntiḥ śāntiḥ śāntiḥ ıı

Om tacchaṁ yorāvṛnīmahe ı gātum yajñāya ı gātum yajñapataye ı daivī swastirastu naḥ ı swastirmānuṣebhyaḥ ı ūrdhvam jigātu bheṣajam ı śan no astu dvipade ı śan catuṣpade ıı Om śāntiḥ śāntiḥ śāntiḥ ıı

Om yaśchandasāmṛṣabho vishvarūpaḥ ı chandobhyo'dhyamṛtāthsambabhūva ı sa mendro medhayā spṛnotu ı amṛtasya devadhārano bhūyāsam ı śarīram me vicarṣaṇam ı jihvā me madhumattamā ı karṇābhyām bhūriviśruvam ı brahmanaḥ kosho'si medhayā pihitaḥ ı śrutam me gopāya ıı Om śāntiḥ śāntiḥ śāntiḥ ıı

Om pūrṇamadaḥ pūrṇamidam pūrṇat pūrṇamudacyate ı pūrṇasya pūrṇamādāya pūrṇamevāvaśiṣyate ıı Om śāntiḥ śāntiḥ śāntiḥ ıı

Om asato mā sadgamaya ı tamaso mā jyotirgamaya ı mrtyormā'mṛtam gamaya ıı Om śāntiḥ śāntiḥ śāntiḥ ıı

## Gayatri Mantra

Om praṇamasya parabrahma ṛṣiḥ paramātmā devatā devī gāyatrī chandaḥ prāṇāyāme viniyogaḥ ıı

Om bhūḥ ı Om bhuvaḥ ı Om suvaḥ ı Om mahaḥ ı Om janaḥ ı Om tapaḥ ı Om satyam ı Om tathsaviturvareṇyam bhargo devasya dhīmahi ı dhiyo yo naḥ pracodayāt ı Om āpo jyothī raso'mṛitam brahma bhūr bhuvaḥ suvarom ıı Om śāntiḥ śāntiḥ śāntiḥ ıı

## Mangala Mantras

Om swasti prajābhyām paripālayantām ।
nyāyena mārgena mahīm mahīśāḥ ।
go brāhmanebhyāśca śubhamastu nityam ।
lokhāh samastā sukhino bhavantu ॥

Sarve jana sukhino bhavantu । samasta sanmaṅgalānisantu । loka kalyāṇa samvṛttirastu viśvaśāntirastu ॥

## Ganesh

Om gaṇānān tvā gaṇapatigm havāmahe kāvin kavīnām upamaśravastamam । jyeṣṭharājam brahmaṇām brahmaṇaspata ā naḥ śṛṇvannūtibhissīda sādanam ॥ Om śrī mahā gaṇapataye namaḥ ॥

Om śuklāmbaradharam viṣṇum śaśivarṇam caturbhujam ।
prasannavadanam dhyāyet sarva vighnopaśāntaye ॥

## Shiva

Om tryambakam yajāmahe sugamdhim puṣṭivardhanam । ūrvārukamiva bandhānmṛtyor mukṣīya mā'mṛtāt ॥Om śāntiḥ śāntiḥ śāntiḥ ॥

## Three Gurus

Om gurur brahmā gurur viṣnuḥ gurur devo maheśvaraḥ ।
guru sākṣāt parabrahma tasmai śrī guruve namaḥ ॥

### Krishna

Jayatu jayatu devo devakī nandoyonam । jayatu jayatu kṛṣṇo vṛṣṇi vamśa pradīpaḥ । jayatu jayatu meghaśyāmlaḥ komalāṅgaḥ । jayatu jayatu kṛṣṇo bhāranāśo mukundaḥ ॥

## Kubera

Om rājādhirājāya prasahyasāhine । namo vayam vaiśravanāya kurmahe । sa me kāmānkāmakāmāyamahyam । kameśvaro vaiśravāṇo dadātu ।
kuberāya vaiśravāṇāya । mahārājāya namaḥ ॥ Om śāntiḥ śāntiḥ śāntiḥ ॥

## Navagra Mantra

Om namaḥ sūryāya candrāya maṅgalāya budhāya ca ।
guruśukraśanibhyāśca rāhuve ketuve nāmaḥ ॥

## Subhashita - Good Sayings

Cintayaścya chittayaścye bindumatra viśuśyate ı cinta dahati nirjivam citta dahati jivanam ॥ Subhaśita

Kāka ahvāyate kākān yaciko na tu yachikān ı kāka yacikormadhye varam kāko na tu yacikaḥ ॥ Subhaśita

## Prayers Goddess in the hand

Kalāgre vasate lakṣmī kalamadye saraswatī ı kalamūle viśālākṣī prabhārte kaladarśanam ॥

## Prayer to rise in the morning

Uttiṣṭhotiṣṭha govinda uttiṣṭha garuḍadhvaja ı uttiṣṭha kamalakaṇṭha trilokyam maṅgalam kuru ॥ 2 ॥

## Prayer to step onto the floor in the morning

Samudre vasne devī parvatastanamaṇḍale ı viṣṇupati nastubhyām pādasparśam kṣamasyame ॥

## For Bad dreams

Rāmaskandham hanumantam vainateyam vṛkodaram ı
śayane yaḥ smaren nityam duḥswapnam tasya naśyati ॥

# CHANTS FROM SHRI SHANKARACHARYA

## The importance of the teacher

Śarīram surūpam tathā vā kalatram ı yaśaścāru citram dhanam merutulyam ı guroraṅghripadme manaścena lagnam tataḥ kim tataḥ kim tataḥ kim tataḥ kim ॥ 1 ॥

## False Teachers

Jaṭalo muṇḍī luñchitakeśaḥ kāṣāyāmbarabahukṛtaveṣaḥ ı
paśyannapi ca na paśyati mūḍho hyudaranimittan bahukṛtaveṣaḥ ॥ 14

## Samsara

Punarapi jananam punarapi maraṇam punarapi jananījaṭhare śayanam ı
iha samsāre bahudustāre kṛpayā'pāre pāhi murāre ॥ 21 ॥